Small Clinical Trials

Issues and Challenges

Charles H. Evans, Jr., and Suzanne T. Ildstad, *Editors*

Committee on Strategies for Small-Number-Participant
Clinical Research Trials

Board on Health Sciences Policy

INSTITUTE OF MEDICINE

NATIONAL ACADEMY PRESS
Washington, D.C.

NATIONAL ACADEMY PRESS • 2101 Constitution Avenue, N.W. • Washington, DC 20418

NOTICE: The project that is the subject of this report was approved by the Governing Board of the National Research Council, whose members are drawn from the councils of the National Academy of Sciences, the National Academy of Engineering, and the Institute of Medicine. The members of the committee responsible for the report were chosen for their special competences and with regard for appropriate balance.

Support for this project was provided by the National Aeronautics and Space Administration. The views presented in this report are those of the Institute of Medicine Committee on Strategies for Small-Number-Participant Clinical Research Trials and are not necessarily those of the funding agency.

International Standard Book Number 0-309-07333-2

Additional copies of this report are available from the National Academy Press, 2101 Constitution Avenue, N.W., Box 285, Washington, D.C. 20055. Call (800) 624-6242 or (202) 334-3313 (in the Washington metropolitan area), or visit the NAP's home page at **www.nap.edu.** The full text of this report is available at **books.nap.edu/catalog/10078.html.**

For more information about the Institute of Medicine, visit the IOM home page at: **www.iom.edu.**

Printed in the United States of America.

The serpent has been a symbol of long life, healing, and knowledge among almost all cultures and religions since the beginning of recorded history. The serpent adopted as a logotype by the Institute of Medicine is a relief carving from ancient Greece, now held by the Staatliche Museen in Berlin.

First Printing, May 2001
Second Printing, July 2001
Third Printing, October 2001

"Knowing is not enough; we must apply.
Willing is not enough; we must do."

—Goethe

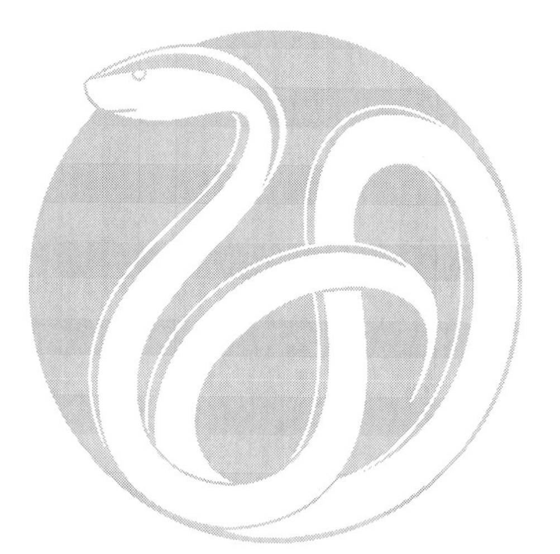

INSTITUTE OF MEDICINE

Shaping the Future for Health

THE NATIONAL ACADEMIES

National Academy of Sciences
National Academy of Engineering
Institute of Medicine
National Research Council

The **National Academy of Sciences** is a private, nonprofit, self-perpetuating society of distinguished scholars engaged in scientific and engineering research, dedicated to the furtherance of science and technology and to their use for the general welfare. Upon the authority of the charter granted to it by the Congress in 1863, the Academy has a mandate that requires it to advise the federal government on scientific and technical matters. Dr. Bruce M. Alberts is president of the National Academy of Sciences.

The **National Academy of Engineering** was established in 1964, under the charter of the National Academy of Sciences, as a parallel organization of outstanding engineers. It is autonomous in its administration and in the selection of its members, sharing with the National Academy of Sciences the responsibility for advising the federal government. The National Academy of Engineering also sponsors engineering programs aimed at meeting national needs, encourages education and research, and recognizes the superior achievements of engineers. Dr. William A. Wulf is president of the National Academy of Engineering.

The **Institute of Medicine** was established in 1970 by the National Academy of Sciences to secure the services of eminent members of appropriate professions in the examination of policy matters pertaining to the health of the public. The Institute acts under the responsibility given to the National Academy of Sciences by its congressional charter to be an adviser to the federal government and, upon its own initiative, to identify issues of medical care, research, and education. Dr. Kenneth I. Shine is president of the Institute of Medicine.

The **National Research Council** was organized by the National Academy of Sciences in 1916 to associate the broad community of science and technology with the Academy's purposes of furthering knowledge and advising the federal government. Functioning in accordance with general policies determined by the Academy, the Council has become the principal operating agency of both the National Academy of Sciences and the National Academy of Engineering in providing services to the government, the public, and the scientific and engineering communities. The Council is administered jointly by both Academies and the Institute of Medicine. Dr. Bruce M. Alberts and Dr. William A. Wulf are chairman and vice chairman, respectively, of the National Research Council.

COMMITTEE ON STRATEGIES FOR SMALL-NUMBER-PARTICIPANT CLINICAL RESEARCH TRIALS

SUZANNE T. ILDSTAD (*Chair*), Director, Institute for Cellular Therapeutics, University of Louisville
ROBERT M. CENTOR, Associate Dean and Director, Division of General Internal Medicine, University of Alabama
ED DAVIS, Professor and Chair, Department of Biostatistics, University of North Carolina School of Public Health, Chapel Hill
BRUCE LEVIN, Professor and Chairman, Division of Biostatistics, The Joseph L. Mailman School of Public Health, Columbia University, New York City
EDWARD D. MILLER, Dean and Chief Executive Officer, The Johns Hopkins University School of Medicine, Baltimore
INGRAM OLKIN, Professor of Statistics and Education, Stanford University, Stanford, CA
DAVID J. TOLLERUD, Professor of Public Health and Director, Center for Environmental and Occupational Health, MCP Hahnemann University School of Public Health, Philadelphia
PETER TUGWELL, Chair, Department of Medicine, University of Ottawa, Ottawa, Canada

Institute of Medicine Board on Health Sciences Policy Liaison

ROBERT D. GIBBONS, Professor of Biostatistics and Director, Center for Health Statistics, University of Illinois at Chicago

Study Staff

CHARLES H. EVANS, JR., Study Director and Senior Adviser, Biomedical and Clinical Research
VERONICA A. SCHREIBER, Research Assistant
TANYA LEE, Project Assistant

Institute of Medicine Staff

ANDREW POPE, Director, Board on Health Sciences Policy
ALDEN CHANG, Administrative Assistant
CARLOS GABRIEL, Financial Associate

Consultant

KATHI E. HANNA

Copy Editor

MICHAEL K. HAYES

Reviewers

The report was reviewed by individuals chosen for their diverse perspectives and technical expertise in accordance with procedures approved by the National Research Council's Report Review Committee. The purpose of this independent review is to provide candid and critical comments to assist the authors and the Institute of Medicine in making the published report as sound as possible and to ensure that the report meets institutional standards for objectivity, evidence, and responsiveness to the study charge. The content of the review comments and the draft manuscript remain confidential to protect the integrity of the deliberative process. The committee wishes to thank the following individuals for their participation in the report review process:

GREGORY CAMPBELL, Director, Division of Biostatistics, Center for Devices and Radiological Health, Food and Drug Administration, Rockville, Maryland
JOSEPH T. COYLE, Chairman, Department of Psychiatry, Harvard Medical School, Boston
NANCY NEVELOFF DUBLER, Director, Division of Bioethics, Montefiore Medical Center, The Albert Einstein College of Medicine, Bronx, New York

LAWRENCE M. FRIEDMAN, Director, Division of Epidemiology and Clinical Applications, National Heart, Lung, and Blood Institute, Bethesda, Maryland
STEVEN N. GOODMAN, Associate Professor, Biostatistics and Medicine, Johns Hopkins University School of Medicine, Baltimore, Maryland
RODERICK LITTLE, Chair, Department of Biostatistics University of Michigan School of Public Health, Ann Arbor, Michigan
DAVID MELTZER, Assistant Professor, Section General Internal Medicine, University of Chicago, Chicago, Illinois
JANE W. NEWBURGER, Director Clinical Research, Children's Hospital, Harvard University, Boston, Massachusetts
RICHARD L. SIMMONS, Medical Director, University of Pittsburgh School of Medicine, Pittsburgh, Pennsylvania
SCOTT L. ZEGER, Chair, Department of Biostatistics, Johns Hopkins University School of Public Health, Baltimore, Maryland

Although the reviewers listed above have provided many constructive comments and suggestions, they were not asked to endorse the conclusions or recommendations nor did they see the final draft of the report before its release. The review of this report was overseen by Joseph T. Coyle, M.D., Chair, Consolidated Department of Psychiatry, Harvard Medical School, Belmont, Massachusetts, who was responsible for making certain that an independent examination of this report was carried out in accordance with institutional procedures and that all review comments were carefully considered. Responsibility for the final content of this report rests entirely with the editors.

Preface

The design and conduct of any type of clinical trial requires three considerations: first, the study should examine valuable and important biomedical research questions; second, it must be based on a rigorous methodology that can answer a specific research question being asked; and third, it must be based on a set of ethical considerations, adherence to which minimizes risks to individuals. Whenever possible standard trial designs should be used in clinical trials. Moreover, investigators should strive to design clinical trials that contain adequate statistical power. However, there are times when the number of experimental subjects is unavoidably small. For example, the rapid progress that is occurring in a variety of areas of science (e.g. biotechnology, organ transplantation, gene therapy, cellular therapies, bioartificial organs, and designer genes tailored to an individual) has resulted in the need for clinical trials with small numbers of participants and new approaches to optimization of the design and analysis of clinical trials when the number of experimental participants (the sample size) in unavoidably small. Clinical trials with small numbers of participants, however, must address broad sets of issues different from those that must be addressed in trials with large numbers of participants. It is in those circumstances of trials with small sample sizes that approaches to optimization of the study design and data interpretation pose greater challenges.

Clinical trials involving astronauts share characteristics with clinical trials of the new technologies mentioned above, as astronauts comprise a population with small numbers of subjects, and many variables that affect this group during space travel cannot be controlled on Earth. However, interventions that prevent potentially life-threatening conditions such as accelerated bone mineral density loss on long space missions must be explored if long missions in space are to be successful. Therefore, the National Aeronautics and Space Administration (NASA) asked the Institute of Medicine (IOM) to convene a panel of experts to recommend optimal approaches to the design, implementation, and evaluation of outcomes in clinical trials with small numbers of participants. NASA commissioned this fast-track study because the opportunity to plan for the next clinical trial during a space mission was rapidly approaching and important questions needed to be answered.

A group of experts in statistics, clinical research study design, epidemiology, and pharmacology made a major effort to prepare what I believe will be a widely useful report. Robert Gibbons, a biostatistician and liaison from the IOM Board on Health Sciences Policy, participated throughout the study as a full committee member. A centerpiece of the committee's activity was an invitational workshop. Experts from the United States and Canada spent a full day providing additional information and expertise to the committee during the invitational workshop discussing future directions for small clinical trials with small numbers of participants. Their efforts were particularly important in helping the committee prepare this report. After careful consideration the committee developed recommendations for approaching the issues and challenges inherent in clinical trials with small sample sizes. Moreover, the design and implementation of future research in this newly developing area of clinical investigation will improve the ability of investigators to evaluate outcomes efficiently and in a cost-effective manner to allow advances in medicine to be available to patients with life-threatening diseases in an efficient manner.

Finally, the IOM staff, led by Charles Evans, contributed significantly to the final outcome. We owe a tremendous gratitude to Kathi Hanna, a highly skilled science writer, and to Veronica Schreiber, the research assistant on the project, for their untiring efforts and assistance to the committee throughout all phases of the study.

Suzanne T. Ildstad
Committee Chair

Contents

Small Clinical Trials

Executive Summary

ABSTRACT

Scientific research has a long history of using well-established, well documented, and validated methods for the design, conduct, and analysis of clinical trials. A study design that is considered appropriate includes sufficient sample size (n) and statistical power and proper control of bias to allow a meaningful interpretation of the results. Whenever feasible, clinical trials should be designed and performed so that they have adequate statistical power. However, when the clinical context does not provide a sufficient number of research participants for a trial with adequate statistical power but the research question has great clinical significance, research can still proceed under certain conditions. Small clinical trials might be warranted for the study of rare diseases, unique study populations (e.g., astronauts), individually tailored therapies, in environments that are isolated, in emergency situations, and in instances of public health urgency. Properly designed trials with small sample sizes may provide substantial evidence of efficacy and are especially appropriate in particular situations. However, the conclusions derived from such studies may require careful consideration of the assumptions and inferences, given the small number of paticipants.

Bearing in mind the statistical power, precision, and validity limitations of trials with small sample sizes, there are innovative design and analysis approaches that can improve the quality of such trials. A number of trial designs especially lend themselves to use in studies with small sample sizes, including one subject (n-of-1) designs, sequential designs, "within-subject" designs, decision analysis-based designs, ranking and selection designs, adaptive designs, and risk-based allocation designs. Data analysis for trials with small numbers of participants in particular must be focused. In general, certain types of analyses are more amenable to studies with small numbers of participants, including sequential analysis, hierarchical analysis, Bayesian analysis, decision analysis, statistical prediction, meta-analysis, and risk-based allocation.

Because of the constraints of conducting research with small sample sizes, the committee makes recommendations in several areas: defining the research question, tailoring the study design by giving careful consideration to alternative methods, clarifying sample characteristics and methods for the reporting of results of clinical trials with small sample sizes, performing corroborative analyses to evaluate the consistency and robustness of the results of clinical trials with small sample sizes, and exercising caution in the interpretation of the results before attempting to extrapolate or generalize the findings of clinical trials with small sample sizes. The committee also recommends that more research be conducted on the development and evaluation of alternative experimental designs and analysis methods for trials with small sample sizes.

INTRODUCTION

Clinical trials are used to elucidate the most appropriate preventive, diagnostic, or treatment options for individuals with a given medical condition. Perhaps the most essential feature of a clinical trial is that it aims to use results based on a limited sample of research participants to see if the intervention is safe and effective or if it is comparable to a comparison treatment. Sample size is a crucial component of any clinical trial. A trial with a small number of research participants is more prone to variability and carries a considerable risk of failing to demonstrate the effectiveness of a given intervention when one really is present. This may occur in phase I (safety and pharmacologic profiles), II (pilot efficacy evaluation), and III (extensive assessment of safety and efficacy) trials. Although phase I and II studies may have smaller sample sizes, they usually have adequate statistical power, which is the committee's definition of a "large" trial. Sometimes a trial with eight participants may have adequate statistical power, statistical power being the probability of rejecting the null hypothesis when the hypothesis is false.

Thus, a critical aspect of clinical trial design is determination of the sample size needed to establish the feasibility of the study (i.e., sufficient statistical power). The number of participants in a clinical trial should always be large enough to provide a sufficiently precise answer to the research question posed, but it should also be the minimum necessary to achieve this aim. A proposed study that cannot answer the question being asked because the necessary sample size cannot be attained should not be conducted on ethical grounds. That is, it is unacceptable to expose patients or research participants to harms even inconveniences if there is no prospect that useful and potentially generalizable information will result from the study.

Adequately powered randomized clinical trials and double-blind, randomized clinical trials are generally regarded as the most authoritative research methods for establishment of the efficacies of therapeutic interventions. By allocating sufficient numbers of individuals to groups (e.g., experimental or control groups), investigators can estimate or determine with some degree of certainty the effect of a given intervention.

Nevertheless, even though the size of the available research population does not allow a randomized clinical trial with adequate statistical power to be conducted, there might still be a need to design and perform the research (e.g., because treatments are unavailable for a rare disorder or a unique patient population or because studies require the participation of patients with terminal or severely debilitating or incapacitating disorders). In addition, some distinctive research populations—such as astronauts or members of a small, isolated community—may consist of less than five individuals. This research situation, in which large numbers of study participants cannot be obtained, is defined as a "small *n* clinical trial," where *n* refers to the sample size. The sample size in small clinical trials might be very small, for example, a group of astronauts during a space mission, or could range upward to more than 100 individuals. This is in contrast to the sample sizes of some large clinical trials, where the number of participants is in the thousands. This report focuses on the issues and challenges presented by clinical trials with very small sample sizes.

Because of the design and analysis constraints of small-sample-size trials and because of their inherent uncertainties, they require at least as much—and probably more—thought and planning than traditional large clinical trials. Small-sample-size studies may also require additional methods for evaluation of the effectiveness of a therapeutic intervention. In addition, inferences should consider the size of the population relative to the size of the sample. For example, in some trials with small sample sizes, the size of the potential population might be large (e.g., phase II studies of treatments for cancer). In other cases, the sample size is necessarily small by virtue of the limited available population (e.g., astronauts). Designs focused on individual effects, such as *n*-of-1 studies seem more appropriate when the available population is limited than when the size of the potential population is large. Sampling of small populations is a problem in its own right and is distinct from the problem of making inferences (extrapolations) from the results of studies with small sample sizes. A threshold question, however, is whether the scientific bases of alternative and emerging methods, such as decision analysis or statistical prediction, alone or in combination, are sufficiently developed to demonstrate the efficacy or effectiveness of a therapeutic intervention in a small clinical trial.

New approaches to protocol design are needed for studies with small sample sizes that can assess the potential therapeutic efficacies of drugs, biologics, devices, and other medical interventions. The rapid progress that is being made in a variety of areas (e.g., biotechnology, organ transplantation, gene therapy, cell and tissue engineering and therapies, biologically based artificial organs, designer drugs, and space travel) highlights the need to evaluate the effects of experimental interventions so that the benefits that arise from these advances can be made available safely and expeditiously.

CHARGE TO THE COMMITTEE AND PLAN OF ACTION

The Institute of Medicine, at the request of the National Aeronautics and Space Administration, asked a committee of experts to assess the current methodologies and the appropriate situations for the conduct of clinical trials with small sample sizes. The charge included a request to assess the published literature on various strategies such as (1) meta-analysis to combine disparate information from several studies including Bayesian techniques as in the confidence profile method and (2) other alternatives such as assessing therapeutic results in a single treated population (e.g., astronauts) by sequentially measuring whether the intervention is falling above or below a preestablished probability outcome range and meeting predesigned specifications as opposed to incremental improvement.

A committee of nine members comprising experts with knowledge in biostatistics, clinical pharmacology, clinical research, ethics, and research design methods reviewed the scientific literature relevant to clinical trials with small sample sizes and held three meetings, including an invitational conference on future directions in clinical trials with small sample sizes. Conference participants consisted of individuals from federal research and regulatory agencies, industry, academia, and other areas of clinical research and practice. They were asked to provide information and perspective on the progress in developing strategies for the design, conduct, and evaluation of clinical trials with small sample sizes.

FINDINGS

- Scientific research has a long history of using well-established, documented, and validated methods for the design, conduct, and analysis of clinical trials (Box 1).
- A study design that is considered appropriate includes one with a sufficient sample size and statistical power and proper control of bias to allow a meaningful interpretation of the results.

The committee strongly reaffirms that, whenever feasible, clinical trials should be designed and performed so that they have adequate statistical power.

- However, when the clinical context does not provide a sufficient number of research participants for a trial with an adequate statistical power but the research question has great clinical significance, research can still proceed under certain conditions.
- Properly designed trials with small sample sizes can contribute to substantial evidence of efficacy and are especially appropriate in particular situations (Box 2). However, the conclusions derived from such studies may require careful consideration of the assumptions and inferences, given the

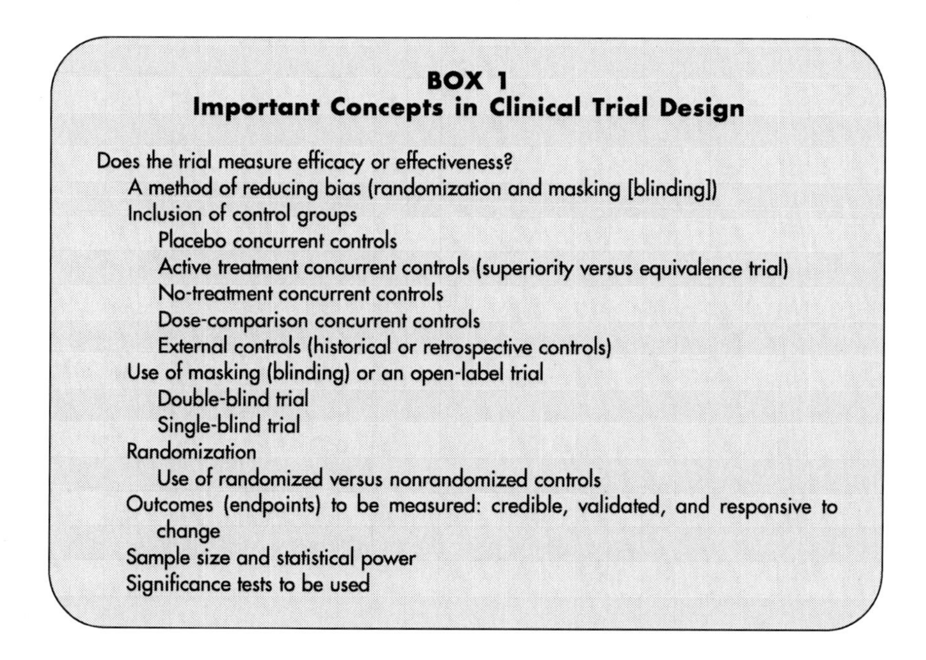

BOX 1
Important Concepts in Clinical Trial Design

Does the trial measure efficacy or effectiveness?
- A method of reducing bias (randomization and masking [blinding])
- Inclusion of control groups
  - Placebo concurrent controls
  - Active treatment concurrent controls (superiority versus equivalence trial)
  - No-treatment concurrent controls
  - Dose-comparison concurrent controls
  - External controls (historical or retrospective controls)
- Use of masking (blinding) or an open-label trial
  - Double-blind trial
  - Single-blind trial
- Randomization
  - Use of randomized versus nonrandomized controls
- Outcomes (endpoints) to be measured: credible, validated, and responsive to change
- Sample size and statistical power
- Significance tests to be used

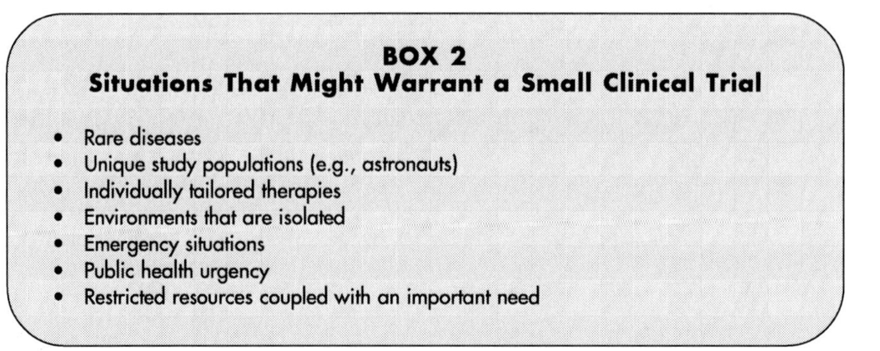

BOX 2
Situations That Might Warrant a Small Clinical Trial

- Rare diseases
- Unique study populations (e.g., astronauts)
- Individually tailored therapies
- Environments that are isolated
- Emergency situations
- Public health urgency
- Restricted resources coupled with an important need

paucity of data. There is nothing very different about small clinical trials relative to larger clinical trials other than greater uncertainty about the inferences made from the results of the trials.

Design and Analysis of Small Clinical Trials

Bearing in mind the statistical power, precision, and validity limitations of trials with small sample sizes, the committee notes that there are innovative design and analysis approaches that can improve the quality of such trials.

A number of trial designs especially lend themselves to use in studies with small sample sizes, including *n*-of-1 designs, sequential designs, decision analysis-based designs, ranking and selection designs, adaptive designs, and risk-based allocation designs (Box 3).

A necessary companion to a well-designed clinical trial is an appropriate statistical analysis of the data from that trial. Assuming that a clinical trial will produce data that could reveal differences in effect between two or more interventions, statistical analyses are used to determine whether such differences are real or due to chance. Analysis of data from trials with small sample sizes in particular must be focused. In general, certain types of analyses are more amenable to trials with small sample sizes (Box 4). Analysis should include confidence intervals when appropriate, although in trials with small sample sizes the confidence intervals will often be uninformative because they will be too wide.

Although Bayesian methods require the use of subjective prior distributions, in small trials it will often be possible to use data from other sources to define the prior distributions. For example, for the problem of loss of bone mineral density during spaceflight, data from earlier spaceflights and studies

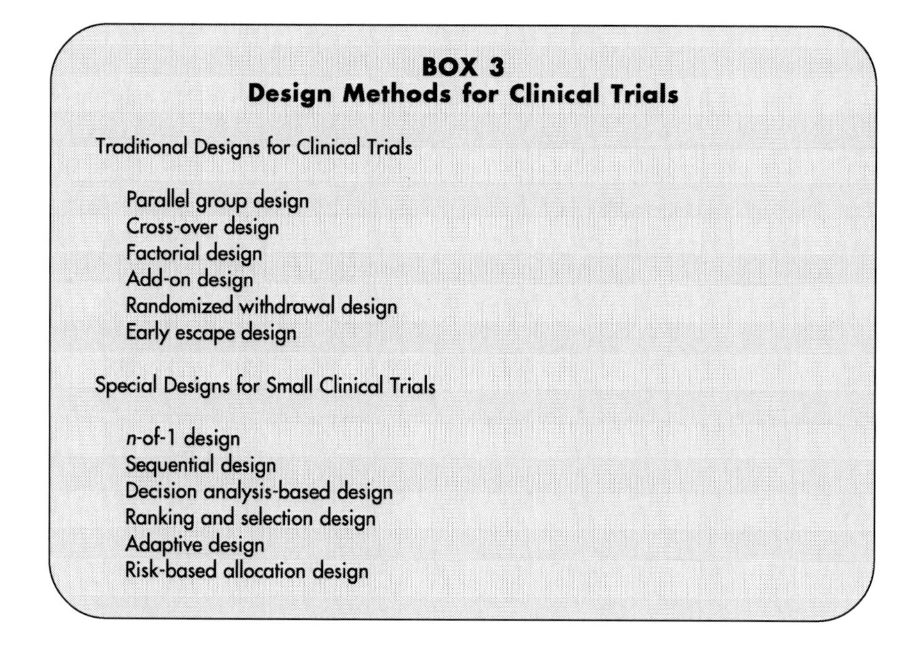

BOX 3
Design Methods for Clinical Trials

Traditional Designs for Clinical Trials

Parallel group design
Cross-over design
Factorial design
Add-on design
Randomized withdrawal design
Early escape design

Special Designs for Small Clinical Trials

n-of-1 design
Sequential design
Decision analysis-based design
Ranking and selection design
Adaptive design
Risk-based allocation design

of osteoporosis in immobilized individuals could provide a strong basis for development of prior distributions. These prior distributions could be used in a sequential trial setting that uses Bayesian methods, which would possibly add considerably to the power of the study.

RECOMMENDATIONS

Because of the constraints of trials with small sample sizes, for example, trials with participants with unique or rare diseases or health conditions, it is

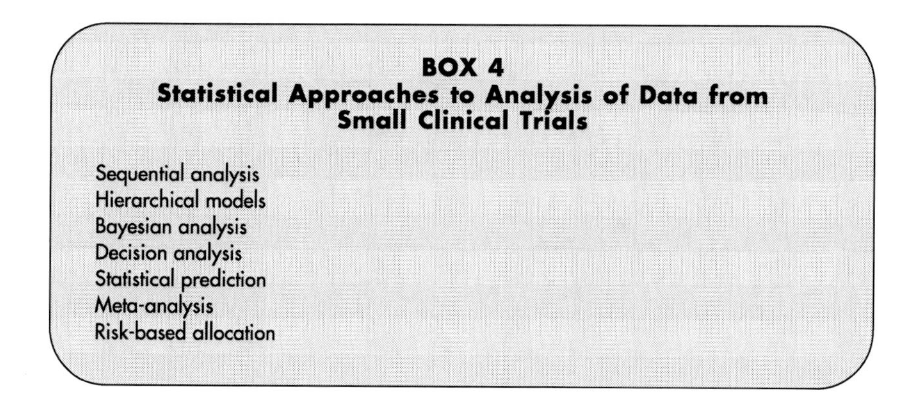

BOX 4
Statistical Approaches to Analysis of Data from Small Clinical Trials

Sequential analysis
Hierarchical models
Bayesian analysis
Decision analysis
Statistical prediction
Meta-analysis
Risk-based allocation

particularly important to define the research questions and select outcome measures that will make the best possible use of the available research participants while minimizing the risks to those participants. The limitations of small trials make it especially important that intermediate and surrogate outcomes be considered for measurement. It will not always be possible to measure directly the effect of an intervention on a given condition.

RECOMMENDATION 1: Define the research question. Before undertaking a small clinical trial it is particularly important that the research question be well defined and that the outcomes and conditions to be evaluated be selected in a manner that will most likely help clinicians make therapeutic decisions.

A multidisciplinary team of experts should be assembled to plan the research effort prospectively. Planning of clinical trials is a multistep process, and alternative methods should be considered to identify the most meaningful answer. To ensure that all approaches and limitations are considered, individuals experienced in trial design, statistics, and medicine are needed during the development of the research plan.

In general, a small clinical trial is conducted because of external constraints, not necessarily by choice. Nonetheless, the common requirements for these trials should be no different from those for larger trials; that is, they must be soundly designed and appropriately analyzed to provide a reasonable measure of the effect of an intervention. They should be designed to have an outcome measure for determination of success, a baseline for the measurement of change, and a means to follow up the study participants to assess change.

RECOMMENDATION 2: Tailor the design. Careful consideration of alternative statistical design and analysis methods should occur at all stages in the multistep process of planning a clinical trial. When designing a small clinical trial, it is particularly important that the statistical design and analysis methods be customized to address the clinical research question and study population.

Because of the limitations of small clinical trials, it is especially important that the results be reported with accompanying details about the sample size, sample characteristics, and study design. The details necessary to combine evidence from several related studies, for example, measurement methods, main outcomes, and predictors for individual participants should be published. There are two reasons for this: first, it allows the clinician to interpret appropriately the data within the clinical context; second, it paves the way for future analyses of the study, for example, as part of a sequential design or a meta-analysis. In the clinical setting, the consequences might be greater if one misinterprets the results. In the research setting, insufficiently described design strategies and methods diminish the study's value for future analyses.

> **RECOMMENDATION 3: Clarify methods of reporting of results of clinical trials. In reporting the results of a small clinical trial, with its inherent limitations, it is particularly important to carefully describe all sample characteristics and methods of data collection and analysis for synthesis of the data from the research.**

Since analysis of the data from small clinical trials will inevitably involve a number of assumptions, the use of several different statistical analyses is likely to enhance the acceptance (or rejection) of various assumptions. For example, if several different analyses give consistent results under different assumptions, one can be more confident that the results are not due to unwarranted assumptions. Conversely, if the analyses produce different results, depending on which sets of assumptions are used, one might be less certain about the original assumptions than might have been the case before the trial was conducted. In sum, the use of alternative statistical analyses might help identify the more sensitive variables and the key interactions in applying heterogeneous results across trials or in trying to draw generalizations from a number of trials.

> **RECOMMENDATION 4: Perform corroborative statistical analyses. Given the greater uncertainties inherent in small clinical trials, several alternative statistical analyses should be performed to evaluate the consistency and robustness of the results of a small clinical trial.**

In small clinical trials, more so than in large clinical trials, one must be particularly cautious about recognizing individual variability among participants in terms of their biology and health care preferences and administrative variability in terms of what can be done from one setting to another. The diminished power of studies with small sample sizes might mean that the generalizability of the findings might not be a possibility in the short term, if at all. Thus, caution should be exercised in the interpretation of the results of small clinical trials.

RECOMMENDATION 5: Exercise caution in interpretation. One should exercise caution in the interpretation of the results of small clinical trials before attempting to extrapolate or generalize those results.

Researchers who participate in clinical trials have proposed alternative clinical trial designs, some of which have been applied to small clinical trials. The committee believes that the research base in this area requires further development. Alternative designs have been proposed in a variety of contexts; however, they have not been adequately examined in the context of small clinical trials. Studies of the use and effectiveness of various designs should be conducted and new methods should be developed. Evaluations of the utilities of individual and combined statistical analyses in a variety of small clinical trial designs will be necessary.

RECOMMENDATION 6: More research on alternative designs is needed. Appropriate federal agencies should increase support for expanded theoretical and empirical research on the performances of alternative study designs and analysis methods that can be applied to small studies. Areas worthy of more study may include theory development, simulated and actual testing including comparison of existing and newly developed or modified alternative designs and methods of analysis, simulation models, study of limitations of trials with different sample sizes, and modification of a trial during its conduct.

CONCLUDING REMARKS

It should be noted that the various strategies and methodologies presented in this report are by no means an exhaustive list of those methods that are applicable to small clinical trials. Indeed, other strategies may be useful on a case-by-case basis. Moreover, the committee believes that all of the strategies described here have potential utility in specific settings and in studies with particular research characteristics and challenges. As a result, no single approach is advocated above all others. In addition, this is a developing area of research. New approaches to this problem will surely arise in the future and may well be in progress.

The importance of conducting small clinical trials only when there are no alternatives cannot be overemphasized. The committee is not encouraging the use of small clinical trials, but, rather provides advice on strategies that should be considered in the design and analysis of small clinical trials when the opportunity to perform a randomized clinical trial with adequate statistical power is not possible. In doing so, it recognizes that small clinical trials frequently need to be viewed as part of a continuing process of data collection. Thus, for some trials it might be impossible to definitively answer a research question with a high degree of confidence. In those cases, perhaps the best that one can do is assess the next set of questions to be asked.

SUMMARY OF THE COMMITTEE'S RECOMMENDATIONS

RECOMMENDATION 1: Define the research question. Before undertaking a small clinical trial it is particularly important that the research question be well defined and that the outcomes and conditions to be evaluated be selected in a manner that will most likely help clinicians make therapeutic decisions.

RECOMMENDATION 2: Tailor the design. Careful consideration of alternative statistical design and analysis methods should occur at all stages in the multistep process of planning a clinical trial. When designing a small clinical trial, it is particularly important that the statistical design and analysis methods be customized to address the clinical research question and study population.

RECOMMENDATION 3: Clarify methods of reporting the results of clinical trials. In reporting the results of a small clinical trial, with its inherent limitations, it is particularly important to carefully describe all sample characteristics and methods of data collection and analysis for synthesis of the data from the research.

RECOMMENDATION 4: Perform corroborative statistical analyses. Given the greater uncertainties inherent in small clinical trials, several alternative statistical analyses should be performed to evaluate the consistency and robustness of the results of a small clinical trial.

RECOMMENDATION 5: Exercise caution in interpretation. One should exercise caution in the interpretation of the results of small clinical trials before attempting to extrapolate or generalize those results.

RECOMMENDATION 6: More research on alternative designs is needed. Appropriate federal agencies should increase support for expanded theoretical and empirical research on the performances of alternative study designs and analysis methods that can be applied to small studies. Areas worthy of more study may include theory development, simulated and actual testing including comparison of existing and newly developed or modified alternative designs and methods of analysis, simulation models, study of limitations of trials with different sample sizes, and modification of a trial during its conduct.

1
Introduction

In the past several decades there has been exponential growth in the number of clinical trials conducted to test innovations in the treatment of disease. A search of the 1999 Medline database alone found reports of 19,587 such trials (Meinert, 2000). In addition, in the past 10 years clinical trials of drugs and other interventions have become more than a process required to judge the safeties and efficacies of potential treatments. They

BOX 1-1
What Is a Clinical Trial?

A clinical trial is defined as a prospective study comparing the effect and value of intervention(s) against control in human beings (Friedman, Furberg, and DeMets, 1996).

A controlled experiment having a clinical event as an outcome measure and done in a clinic or clinical setting and involving persons having a specific disease or health condition (Meinert, 1996).

An experiment is a series of observations made under conditions controlled by the scientist. A clinical trial is an experiment testing medical treatments on human participants (Piantadosi, 1997).

The term clinical trials may be applied to any form of planned experiment which involves patients and is designed to elucidate the most appropriate treatment of future patients with a given medical condition (Pocock, 1984).

have also become part of the health care system, in that patients often view participation in a clinical trial as their best hope of achieving a cure (Zivin, 2000).

Although there are different interpretations of the term "clinical trial," in general, it is defined as an experiment designed to assess the safety or efficacy of a test treatment (Meinert, 2000) (Box 1-1). Clinical trials refer to planned experiments that involve human participants and that are designed to elucidate the most appropriate treatments for future patients with a given medical condition (Pocock, 1984). Perhaps the most essential feature of a clinical trial is that it aims to use results for a limited sample of patients to make inferences about how treatment should be administered to the general population of patients who will require therapy in the future (Pocock, 1984).

WHEN THE STANDARD APPROACH TO CLINICAL TRIALS IS NOT FEASIBLE

Adequately powered randomized clinical trials (RCTs) and double blind RCTs are generally regarded as the most authoritative research methods for establishment of the efficacies of therapeutic interventions. By allocating sufficient numbers of individuals to groups—for example, an experimental or a control group—investigators can estimate or determine with some degree of certainty the effect of a given intervention.

However, when the available population of research participants does not allow the conduct of an RCT with adequate statistical power, there might still be a need to design and perform clinical research (e.g., treatments are not available for a rare disorder or a unique patient population or studies require the participation of patients with terminal or severely debilitating or incapacitating disorders). Some distinctive research populations—such as astronauts or members of a small, isolated community—may consist of less than five individuals. For example, a study focused on assessing the effects of microgravity on bone mineral density loss during space missions would have to rely on data for a few individuals (see Box 1-2). This report defines this research situation as a *small clinical trial* and explores the various design and analytical strategies one might consider to approach a small clinical trial.

Obtaining sufficiently large control groups for research with small numbers of participants can be difficult for research involving individuals with severe, debilitating, or incapacitating conditions, and the use of untreated or placebo control groups can raise ethical dilemmas (Altman, 2000; Delaney, 2000; Emond, 2000). Historically, drug developers and federal regulators have been wary of small clinical trials for a number of reasons, but primarily

BOX 1-2
Case Study: Effects of Long-Term Microgravity Exposure on Weight-Bearing Bones of Cosmonauts

Microgravity-induced bone mineral density (BMD) loss was first suspected in the 1970s, but systematic investigations with astronauts and cosmonauts did not commence until the 1990s. Investigation is made difficult because there are few potential participants and the conditions of microgravity, in terms of length of exposure, vary with the lengths of space missions and the availability of individual astronauts or cosmonauts to participate in clinical investigations while they are on those missions.

Observational studies suggest that the loss in BMD may be on the order of 1 to 2 percent per month during extended exposure to microgravity. Recently, Vico et al. (2000) reported measurements of BMD at the distal radius and tibia in 15 cosmonauts on the Russian *Mir* space station who had sojourned in space for 1 month ($n = 2$), 2 months ($n = 2$), or 6 months ($n = 11$) since 1994. BMD was measured before launch and the week after landing. Each cosmonaut who spent at least 2 months in space was allowed a recovery period equal to the duration of the corresponding space mission.

The findings demonstrate striking interindividual variations in BMD responses and indicated that the BMD of neither cancellous bone nor cortical bone of the radius was significantly changed at any time. In the weight-bearing tibial site, however, cancellous BMD loss was already present after the first month and deteriorated with mission duration. In tibial corticies, BMD loss was noted after a 2-month mission. In the group who had been in space for 6 months, cortical BMD loss was less pronounced than cancellous BMD loss. In some individuals the tibial BMD deterioration was marked. Variations in tibial BMD loss were also large during recovery, and the loss persisted in some individuals. These studies have found a mean BMD loss of about 2 percent after 6 months of space travel, with a standard deviation of approximately 1.2 percent. If the clinically important effect of an intervention that limits the total BMD loss to 1 percent is to be detected, the total sample size needed is 50 (significance level = 5 percent with power of 90 percent [as determined by a one-sided *t* test]). With only three to six astronauts per flight and one or two long missions per year, it would take up to 10 years to evaluate a single intervention in a traditional clinical trials.

The challenge is to conduct clinical trials with small populations to evaluate the efficacies of various interventions for the prevention of BMD.

because of their lack of statistical power and generalizability (Table 1-1). Thus, in general, a small clinical trial is conducted because of external constraints, not necessarily by choice. Nonetheless, the general requirements for small clinical trials are no different than those for adequately powered "large clinical" trials; that is, they must be sufficiently designed and appropriately analyzed to provide a reasonable measure of the effect of an intervention. They should be designed to have an outcome measure for determination of success, a baseline measure that can be used to determine changes, and a means to monitor the changes (Meinert, 2000). Because of the design

TABLE 1-1 Concerns About Small Clinical Trials

- Small numbers leave much to chance.
- Statistically significant outcomes from small clinical trials may not be as generalizable because the circumstances in which the rules apply may be narrower than those for larger clinical studies with identical probabilities (*p* values).
- Often, there are too many variables to ascertain cause and effect to any meaningful degree.
- Small clinical trials are unlikely to tease out anything but gross effects and are limited in their ability to analyze covariates.
- For studies of drugs, and other interventions, small clinical trials may be incapable of identifying true side effects and safety concerns and are also constrained for the reasons listed above.

SOURCE: Delaney (2000).

and analysis constraints of small clinical trials and because of uncertainties inherent to small clinical trials, it is likely that they will require at least as much—and probably more—thought than traditional, large clinical trials.

In some cases, however, properly designed small clinical trials can contribute to substantial evidence of efficacy; however, those conclusions may require the use of assumptions and inferences given the paucity of data (Siegel, 2000). Small clinical trials may successfully be used to study diseases or conditions with a well-described natural history with little variation; when sensitive pharmacodynamic effects are directly related to pathophysiology; when good nonhuman models are available; and when the intervention has a large effect on efficacy, produces a predictable relationship between measurable drug levels and effects, and has been applied to a related condition (Siegel, 2000) (Table 1-2). Traditionally, small studies are more likely to be conducted to test surgical procedures than to test drugs (Delaney, 2000; Emond, 2000) (Box 1-3). They are least likely to be useful for the study of complex disease syndromes with highly variable outcomes (e.g., some chronic diseases such as arteriosclerotic cardiovascular disease), for drugs with less than dramatic effects in vitro, for illnesses in which correlates of success are unclear, in situations in which the risk of short-term death is high, and for surgical procedures for which there are many complex and confounding factors (Delaney, 2000; Faustman, 2000; Mishoe, 2000).

A SEARCH FOR ALTERNATIVES

New approaches to protocol design are needed for trials with small sample sizes that can assess the potential therapeutic efficacies of drugs,

TABLE 1-2 Situations That Might Warrant a Small Clinical Trial

- Rare diseases
- Unique study populations (e.g., astronauts)
- Individually tailored therapies
- Environments that are remote or isolated
- Emergency situations
- Public health urgency
- Restricted resources coupled with a high level of need

biologics, devices, and other medical interventions. For example, a possible alternative is to assess the therapeutic results in a single treated population by sequentially measuring whether the intervention results in outcomes that

BOX 1-3
Case Study: Clinical Trial of Organ Transplantation in HIV-Positive Individuals

Human immunodeficiency virus (HIV)-positive individuals now live long enough to be considered candidates for cardiac or liver transplantation (Gow and Mutimer, 2001). A very small number of HIV-positive organs become available for transplantation into HIV-positive individuals. Whether the immunosuppressive agents required for organ transplantation will accelerate or slow the progression of HIV infection or AIDS is an unresolved research question. A study is underway to evaluate the outcomes of transplants of hearts and livers from HIV-positive donors into HIV-positive recipients. There are a small number of candidates for such a study, and the only alternative is to not do a transplant. In that event, death is the ultimate outcome since long-term alternative supports—for example, dialysis for renal failure—are not available for patients with liver failure.

The research question to be answered in a clinical trial is whether transplantation will benefit patients with HIV infection or AIDS with a diminished life expectancy from cardiac or liver failure due to their impaired organs if they do not receive a transplant? The ideal study should determine the risk of transplantation (and associated interventions) on the progression of HIV infection or AIDS and its effect on life expectancy. The projected life expectancy is approximately 6 months without transplantation, and only 5 percent of the participants are expected to be alive after 12 months. The 1-year survival rate after standard heart and liver transplantation in non-HIV infected individuals approaches 90 percent. A survival rate of 25 percent at 1 year in the HIV-infected or AIDS patients who receive a transplant would be a clinically important advance. With a significance level of 0.05 and a power of 0.9, the sample size needed to detect an increase in the 1-year survival rate from 5 to 25 percent is 150. At the current rate of organ availability, such a study would take many years.

fall above or below a preestablished probability range for an efficacious outcome. Such a clinical trial could be considered to have demonstrated efficacy when the cumulative observed results fall within or above the prescribed confidence range, or the trial could be stopped when the cumulative observed effect falls below the preestablished level of confidence (Box 1-4). A major question, however, for this and other approaches is whether the science base of alternative methods alone or in combination is sufficiently developed for these nonrandomized clinical trials to be effective in demonstrating efficacy in studies with small sample size.

It has been recognized for some time that RCTs—although highly desirable—are neither practical nor feasible as a means of answering all clinical research questions. A variety of other methods, such as non-RCTs, observational methods, naturalistic studies, and case-control studies, have been used in clinical investigations. In addition, there has been increasing discussion over the past decade about the value of measuring surrogate markers rather than traditional clinical endpoints in clinical trials.

BOX 1-4
Case Study: Clinical Trial for Treatment of Sickle Cell Disease

Sickle cell disease is a red blood cell (RBC) disorder that affects 1 in 200 African Americans. Half of all individuals living with sickle cell disease die before age 40. The most common complications include stroke, renal failure, and chronic severe pain. Patients who have a stroke are predisposed to having another one.

Mixed donor and host stem cell chimerism (i.e., the sickle cell host recipient has a cellular constitution made up of both the donor and the recipient subject's cells) is curative for sickle cell disease (Krishnamutri, Blazar, and Wagner, 2001). Only 20 percent donor RBC production (with 80 percent recipient RBC production) is required to cure the abnormality. Conditioning of the recipient is required for the bone marrow transplant to be successfully established. The degree of human leukocyte antigen (HLA) mismatch, as well as the sensitization state (i.e., chronic transfusion immunizes the recipient), influences how much conditioning is required to establish 20 percent donor chimerism.

In patients who have an HLA-identical donor and who have not been heavily transfused, 200 centigrays of total body irradiation (TBI) is sufficient to establish donor engraftment. This dose of irradiation has been shown to be safe and well tolerated. In heavily transfused recipients who are HLA-mismatched, more conditioning will probably be required. The optimal dose of TBI for this cohort has not been established. The focus of this hypothetical study is to establish the optimum dose of TBI dose to achieve 20 percent donor chimerism in patients enrolled in the protocol (Chapter 3).

In 1990, the Institute of Medicine (IOM) published *Medical Intervention at the Crossroads: Modern Methods of Clinical Investigation*, which discussed the benefits and drawbacks of non-RCTs. However, the issue of when and how to conduct a small clinical trial continues to challenge many areas of biomedical science.

IOM COMMITTEE PROCESS AND STATEMENT OF TASK

In response to the growing need for reliable and valid methods for clinical research with small populations, the National Aeronautics and Space Administration requested that the IOM undertake a study of strategies for small-number-participant clinical research trials. However, the term "small number" may convey different meanings to different constituencies; consequently, the committee prefers to use the phrase "small clinical studies" or "small clinical trials."

The committee, consisting of individuals with expertise in biostatistics, clinical pharmacology, clinical research, ethics, and research design, was charged with the following specific tasks:

- Assess the current methodologies for conducting clinical trials with small populations. The analysis of methods used to conduct small clinical trials will include assessment of the published literature and commissioned papers on various strategies such as (1) meta-analysis to combine disparate information from several studies, including Bayesian techniques, as in the confidence profile method, and (2) other alternatives to RCTs, such as assessments of therapeutic results for a single treated population by sequentially measuring whether the outcomes from the intervention fall above or below a preestablished probability outcome range and meet predesigned specifications as opposed to incremental improvements.
- Convene a 1-day conference during which participants from federal research and regulatory agencies, industry, academia, and other areas of clinical research and practice will discuss the progress being made in the strategies and the state of the science in the design, conduct, and evaluation of clinical trials of drugs, biologics, devices, and other medical interventions in populations with small numbers of individuals. Methods including RCTs, meta-analysis, decision analysis, and sequential clinical trial approaches will be considered in terms of their potentials and problems. The discussions will include, where possible, ethical and statistical evaluations and comparisons.

• The committee, through consideration of background materials and presentations at the conference, will review the methodology for clinical trials with small populations and make recommendations for future research to continue development of this area of medical research.

ORGANIZATION OF THE REPORT

This report is organized around the two major issues in the performance of any clinical trial: design and analysis. Chapter 2 addresses the fundamental tenets of clinical trial design and how they are challenged and possibly addressed by studies with small numbers of participants. Chapter 3 focuses on several statistical approaches that can be used to analyze small clinical trials. Each chapter provides recommendations and suggests research needs.

It should be noted that the various strategies and methodologies presented in this report are by no means an exhaustive list of those methods that are applicable to small clinical trials. Indeed, other strategies not presented here may be useful on a case-by-case basis. Moreover, this is a developing area of research, and new approaches to small clinical trials will arise in the future and may well be in progress. Finally, the amount of attention paid to a particular area described in the report is not necessarily proportional to its importance or utility but, rather, may have been motivated by a particular example that the committee used to illustrate a small-sample-size clinical problem and potential solution. The committee's goal is to provide a balanced overview and analysis of various methods in use and to suggest new ones where appropriate.

2
Design of Small Clinical Trials

The design and conduct of any type of clinical trial require three considerations: first, the study should examine valuable and important biomedical research questions; second, it must be based on a rigorous methodology that can answer a specific research question being asked; and third, it must be based on a set of ethical considerations, adherence to which minimizes the risks to the study participants (Sutherland, Meslin, and Till, 1994). The choice of an appropriate study design depends on a number of considerations, including:

- the ability of the study design to answer the primary research question;
- whether the trial is studying a potential new treatment for a condition for which an established, effective treatment already exists;
- whether the disease for which a new treatment is sought is severe or life-threatening;
- the probability and magnitude of risk to the participants;
- the probability and magnitude of likely benefit to the participants;
- the population to be studied—its size, availability, and accessibility; and
- how the data will be used (e.g., to initiate treatment or as preliminary data for a larger trial).

Because the choice of a study design for any particular trial will depend on these and other factors, no general prescription can be offered for the design of clinical trials. However, certain key issues are raised when randomized clinical trials (RCTs) with adequate statistical power are not feasible and when studies with smaller populations must be considered. The utility of such studies may be diminished, but not completely lost, and in other ways may be enhanced.

To understand what is lost or gained in the design and conduct of studies with very small numbers of participants, it is important to first consider the basic tenets of clinical trial design (Box 2-1).

KEY CONCEPTS IN CLINICAL TRIAL DESIGN

Judgments about the effectiveness of a given intervention ultimately rest on an interpretation of the strength of the evidence arising from the data collected. In general, the more controlled the trial, the stronger is the evidence.

The study designs for clinical trials can take several forms, most of which are based on an assumption of accessible sample populations. Clinical trials of efficacy ask whether the experimental treatment works under ideal condi-

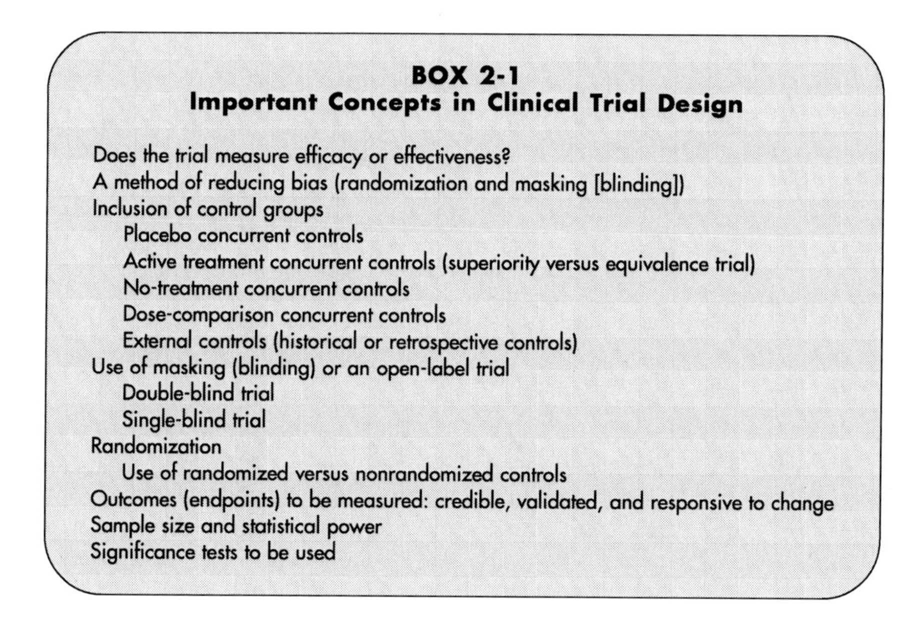

BOX 2-1
Important Concepts in Clinical Trial Design

Does the trial measure efficacy or effectiveness?
A method of reducing bias (randomization and masking [blinding])
Inclusion of control groups
- Placebo concurrent controls
- Active treatment concurrent controls (superiority versus equivalence trial)
- No-treatment concurrent controls
- Dose-comparison concurrent controls
- External controls (historical or retrospective controls)

Use of masking (blinding) or an open-label trial
- Double-blind trial
- Single-blind trial

Randomization
- Use of randomized versus nonrandomized controls

Outcomes (endpoints) to be measured: credible, validated, and responsive to change
Sample size and statistical power
Significance tests to be used

tions. In contrast, clinical trials of effectiveness ask whether the experimental treatment works under ordinary circumstances. Often, trials of efficacy are not as sensitive to issues of access to care, the generalizability of the results from a study with highly selective sample of patients and physicians, and the level of adherence to treatment regimens. Thus, when a trial of efficacy is done with a small sample of patients, it is not clear whether the experimental intervention will be effective when a broader range of providers and patients use the intervention. On the other hand, trials of effectiveness can be problematic if they produce a negative result, in which case it will be unclear whether the experimental intervention would fail under any circumstances. Thus, the issue of what is preferred in a small clinical study—a trial of efficacy or effectiveness—is an important consideration.

In the United States, the Food and Drug Administration (FDA) oversees the regulation and approval of drugs, biologics, and medical devices. Its review and approval processes affect the design and conduct of most new clinical trials. Preclinical testing of an experimental intervention is performed before investigators initiate a clinical trial. These studies are carried out in the laboratory and in studies with animals to provide preliminary evidence that the experimental intervention will be safe and effective for humans. FDA requires preclinical testing before clinical trials can be started. Safety information from preclinical testing is used to support a request to FDA to begin testing the experimental intervention in studies with humans.

Clinical trials are usually classified into four phases. *Phase I trials* are the earliest-stage clinical trials used to study an experimental drug in humans, are typically small (less than 100 participants), and are often used to determine the toxicity and maximum safe dose of a new drug. They provide an initial evaluation of a drug's safety and pharmacokinetics. Such studies also usually test various doses of the drug to obtain an indication of the appropriate dose to be used in later studies. Phase I trials are commonly conducted with nondiseased individuals (healthy volunteers). Some phase I trials, for example, those of studies of treatments for cancer, are performed with individuals with advanced disease who have failed all other standard treatments (Heyd and Carlin, 1999).

Phase II trials are often aimed at gathering preliminary data on whether a drug has clinical efficacy and usually involve 100 to 300 participants. Frequently, phase II trials are used to determine the efficacy and safety of an intervention in participants with the disease for which a new intervention is being developed.

Phase III trials are advanced-stage clinical trials designed to show conclusively how well a drug works. Phase III trials are usually larger, frequently multi-institutional studies, and typically involve from a hundred to thousands of participants. They are comparative in nature, with participants usually assigned by chance to at least two arms, one of which serves as a control or a reference arm and one or more of which involve new interventions. Phase III trials generally measure whether a new intervention extends survival, or improves the health of participants receiving the intervention and has fewer side effects.

Some phase II and phase III trials are designed as *pivotal trials* (sometimes also called *confirmatory trials*), which are adequately controlled trials in which the hypotheses are stated in advance and evaluated. The goal of a pivotal trial is to attempt to eliminate systematic biases and increase the statistical power of a trial. Pivotal trials are intended to provide firm evidence of safety and efficacy.

Occasionally, FDA requires *phase IV trials*, usually performed after a new drug or biologic has been approved for use. These trials are postmarketing surveillance studies aimed at obtaining additional information about the risks, benefits, and optimal use of an intervention. For example, a phase IV trial may be required by FDA to study the effects of an intervention in a new patient population or for a stage of disease different from that for which it was originally tested. Phase IV trials are also used to assess the long-term effects of an intervention and to reveal rare but serious side effects.

One criticism of the classification of clinical trials presented above is that it focuses on the requirements for the regulation of pharmaceuticals, leaving out the many other medical products that FDA regulates. For example, new heart valves are evaluated by FDA on the basis of their ability to meet predetermined operating performance characteristics. Another device is the intraocular lens whose performance must be satisfied in a prespecified grid. Medical device studies, however, rely on a great deal of information about the behavior of the control group that often cannot be obtained or that is very difficult to obtain in small clinical trials because of the small number or lack of control participants.

A much more inclusive and general approach that subsumes the four phases of clinical trials is put forth by Piantadosi (1997), who defines the four phases as (1) early-development studies (testing the treatment mechanism), (2) middle-development studies (treatment tolerability), (3) comparative (pivotal, confirmatory) studies, and (4) late-development studies (extended safety or postmarketing studies). This approach is more inclusive than trials of pharmaceuticals; it includes trials of vaccines, biological and gene therapies, screening devices, medical devices, and surgical interventions.

The ethical conduct of a clinical study of the benefits of an intervention requires that it begin in a state of *equipoise*. Equipoise is defined as the point at which a rational, informed person—whether patient, provider, or researcher—has no preference between two (or more) available treatments (Freedman, 1987; Lilford and Jackson, 1995). When used in the context of research, equipoise describes a state of genuine uncertainty about whether the experimental intervention offers greater benefit or harm than the control intervention. Equipoise is advocated as a means of achieving high scientific and ethical standards in randomized trials (Alderson, 1996). True equipoise might be more of a challenge in small clinical trials, because the degree of uncertainty might be diminished by the nature of the disorder, the lack of real choices for treatment, or insufficient data to make a judgment about the risks of one treatment arm over another.

A primary purpose of many clinical trials is evaluation of the efficacy of an experimental intervention. In a well-designed trial, the data that are collected and the observations that are made will eventually be used to overturn the equipoise. At the end of a trial, when it is determined whether an experimental intervention has efficacy, the state of clinical equipoise has been eliminated. Central principles in proving efficacy, and thereby eliminating equipoise, are avoiding bias and establishing statistical significance. This is ideally done through the use of controls, randomization, blinding of the study, credible and validated outcomes responsive to small changes, and a sufficient sample size. In some trials, including small clinical studies, the elimination of equipoise in such a straightforward manner might be difficult. Instead, estimation of a treatment effect as precisely as necessary may be sufficient to distinguish the effect from zero. It is a more nuanced approach, but one that should be considered in the study design.

Adherence to an ethical process, whereby risks are minimized and voluntary informed consent is obtained, is essential to any research involving humans and may be particularly acute in small clinical trials, in which the sample population might be easily identified and potentially more vulnerable. Study designs that incorporate an ethical process may help in reducing concerns about some of problems in design and interpretation that naturally accompany small clinical trials.

Reducing Bias

Bias in clinical trials is the potential of any aspects of the design, conduct, analysis, or interpretation of the results of a trial to lead to conclusions about the effects of an intervention that are systematically different from the truth (Pocock, 1984). It is both a scientific and an ethical issue. It is relatively easy to identify potential sources of bias in clinical trials, but investigators have a limited ability to effectively remove the effects of bias. It is often difficult to even determine the net direction and effect of bias on the study results. Randomization and masking (blinding) are the two techniques generally used to minimize bias and to maximize the probability that the test intervention and control groups are similar at the start of the study and are treated similarly throughout its course (Pocock, 1984). Clinical trials with randomized controls and with blinding, when practical and appropriate, represent the standard for the evaluation of therapeutic interventions.

Improper randomization or imperfect masking may result in bias. However, bias may work in any direction (Hauck and Anderson, 1999). In addition, the data for participants who withdraw or are lost from the trial can bias the results.

Alternative Types of Control Groups

A control group in a clinical trial is a group of individuals used as a comparison for a group of participants who receive the experimental treatment. The main purpose of a control group is to permit investigators to determine whether an observed effect is truly caused by the experimental intervention being tested or by other factors, such as the natural progression of the disease, observer or participant expectations, or other treatments (Pocock, 1996). The experience of the control group lets the investigator know what would have happened to study participants if they had not received the test intervention or what would have happened with a different treatment known to be effective. Thus, the control group serves as a baseline.

There are numerous types of control groups, some of which can be used in small clinical trials. FDA classifies clinical trial control groups into five types: *placebo concurrent controls*, *active-treatment concurrent controls*, *no-treatment concurrent controls*, *dose-comparison concurrent controls*, and *external controls* (Food and Drug Administration, 1999). Each type of control group has its strengths and weaknesses, depending on the scientific question being asked, the intervention being tested, and the group of participants involved.

In a trial with *placebo concurrent controls*, the experimental intervention is compared with intervention with a placebo. Participants are randomized to receive either the new intervention or a placebo. Most placebo-controlled trials are also double blind, so that neither the participants nor the physician, investigator, or evaluator knows who is assigned to the placebo group and who will receive the experimental intervention. Placebo-controlled trials also allow a distinction between adverse events due to the intervention and those due to the underlying disease or other potential interference, if they occur sufficiently frequently to be detected with the available sample size. It is generally accepted that a placebo-controlled trial would not be ethical if an established, effective treatment that is known to prevent serious harm, such as death or irreversible injury, is available for the condition being studied (World Medical Association, 1964). There may be some exceptions, however, such as cases in which the established, effective treatment does not work in certain populations or it has such adverse effects that patients refuse therapy. The most recent version of the Declaration of Helsinki (October 2000 [World Medical Association, 2000]) argues that use of a placebo is unethical regardless of the lack of severity of the condition and regardless of whether the best possible treatment is available in the setting or location in which the trial is being conducted. The benefits, risks, burdens, and effectiveness of a new method should be tested against those of the best current prophylactic, diagnostic, and therapeutic methods. At present, many U.S. scientists (including those at FDA) disagree with that point of view. The arguments are complex and need additional discussion and time before a consensus can be achieved if this new direction or another one similar to it is to replace the previous recommendation.

Although placebos are still the most common control used in pharmaceutical trials, it is increasingly common to compare an experimental intervention with an existing established, effective treatment. *Active-treatment concurrent control trials* are extremely useful in cases in which it would not be ethical to give participants a placebo because doing so would pose undue risk to their health or well being. In an active-control study, participants are randomly assigned to the experimental intervention or to an alternative therapy, the active-control treatment. Such trials are usually double blind, but this is not always possible. For example, many oncology studies are considered impossible to blind because of different regimens, different routes of administration, and different toxicities (Heyd and Carlin, 1999). Despite the best intentions, some treatments have unintended effects that are so specific that their occurrence will inevitably identify the treatment received to both the patient and the medical staff. It is particularly important to do everything possible to have blinded interpretation of outcome variables or critical endpoints when the type of treatment is obvious. In a study in which an active control is used, it may be difficult to determine whether any of the treatments has an effect unless the effects of the treatments are obvious or a placebo control is included, or a placebo-controlled trial has previously demonstrated the efficacy of the active control.

Active treatment-controlled trials can take two forms: a *superiority trial*, in which the new drug is evaluated to determine if it is superior to the active control, and an *equivalence trial* (a noninferiority trial), in which the new drug is tested to determine if it is equivalent to but not inferior to the active control (Hauck and Anderson, 1999). Equivalence trials are designed to show that the new intervention is as effective or nearly as effective as the established effective treatment. For diseases for which an established, effective treatment is available and in use, a common design randomizes participants to receive either an experimental intervention or the established, effective treatment. It is not scientifically possible to prove that two different interventions are exactly equivalent, only that they are nearly equivalent.

In a trial with *no-treatment concurrent controls*, a group receiving the experimental intervention is compared with a group not receiving the treatment or placebo. The randomized no-treatment control trial is similar to the placebo-controlled trial. However, since it often cannot be fully blinded, several aspects of the trial may be affected, including retention of participants, patient management, and all aspects of observation (Food and Drug Administration, 1999). A no-treatment concurrent control trial is usually used when blinding is not feasible, such as when a sham surgery would have to be used or when the side effects of the experimental intervention are obvious. No-treatment concurrent control trials can also be used when the effects of the treatment are obvious and there is a small placebo effect. To reduce bias when a no-treatment control is used, it is desirable that those responsible for clinical assessment remain blinded.

In a *dose-comparison concurrent control trial*, participants are assigned to one of several dose groups so that the effects of different doses of the test drug (dose-response) can be compared. Most dose-response-controlled trials are randomized and double blind. They may include a placebo group or an active control group or both. For example, it is not uncommon to show no difference between doses in a dose-response study. Unless the action of the drug is obvious, inclusion of a placebo group is extremely useful to determine if the drug being tested has no effect at all or a constant positive effect above the minimum dose.

There are several advantages to using a dose-response control instead of a placebo control. When an experimental intervention has pharmacological effects that could break the blinding, it may be easier to preserve blinding in a dose-response study than in a placebo-controlled trial (Food and Drug Administration, 1999). Also, if the optimally safe and effective dose of an experimental intervention is not known, it may be more useful to study a range of doses than to choose a single dose that may be suboptimal or toxic (Pocock, 1996). Sometimes the optimal dose of a drug has unacceptable toxicity and a lower dose—even though it is not optimal for the treatment of the disease—is safer. In this case, a dose-response-controlled trial can be used to optimize the effective dose while minimizing the concomitant toxicity. However, the same ethical issues related to withholding an established, effective treatment from participants in placebo-controlled trials are relevant in a dose-response study (Clark and Leaverton, 1994).

In an *external control trial*, participants receiving the intervention being tested are compared with a group of individuals who are separate from the population tested in the trial. The most common type of external control is a *historical control* (sometimes called a *retrospective control*) (Gehan, 1982). Individuals receiving the experimental intervention are compared with a group of individuals tested at an earlier time. For example, the results of a prior clinical trial published in the medical literature may serve as a historical control. The major problem with historical controls is that one cannot ensure that the comparison is fair because of the variability in patient selection and the experimental environment. If historical controls are obtained from a previous trial conducted in the same environment or by the same investigators, there is a greater chance of reducing the potential bias (Pocock, 1984). Studies have shown that externally controlled trials tend to overestimate the efficacies of experimental treatments (Sacks, Chalmers, and Smith, 1982), although one example has found the treatment effect to be underestimated (Farewell and D'Angio, 1981). Therefore, when selecting an external control, it is extremely important to try to control for these biases by selecting the control group before testing of the experimental intervention and ensuring that the control group is similar to the experimental group in as many ways as possible.

Trials with external controls sometimes compare the group receiving the experimental intervention with a group tested during the same time period but in another setting. A variation of an externally controlled trial is a *baseline-controlled trial* (e.g., a before-or-after trial). In a baseline-controlled trial, the health condition of the individuals before they received the experimental intervention is compared with their condition after they have received the intervention.

It is increasingly common for studies to have more than one type of control group, for example, both an active control and a placebo control. In those trials the placebo control serves as an internal control to provide evidence that the active control had an effect. Some trials compare several doses of a test drug with several doses of an active control drug, all of which may then be compared with a placebo.

In some instances, the only practical way to design a clinical trial is as an *uncontrolled trial.* Uncontrolled trials are usually used to test new experimental interventions for diseases for which no established, effective treatments are available and the prognosis is universally poor without therapy. In uncontrolled trials, there is no control group for comparison, and it is not possible to use blinding and randomization to minimize bias. Uncontrolled trials are similar to externally controlled trials, in the sense that the outcomes for research participants receiving the experimental intervention are compared with the outcomes before the availability of the intervention. Therefore, the scientific grounds for the experimental intervention must be strong enough and its effects must be obvious enough for the positive results of an uncontrolled trial to be accepted. History is replete with examples of failed uncontrolled trials, such as those for the drug laetrile and the anticancer agent interferon (Pocock, 1984).

Matching and Stratification

In many cases investigators may be faced with a situation in which they have a potentially large historical control sample that they want to compare with a small experimental sample in terms of one or more endpoints. This is typically a problem in observational studies in which the individuals have not been randomized to the control and experimental groups. The question is, how does one control for the bias inherent in the observational nature of these data? Perhaps the experimental participants have in some way been self-selected for their illness or the intervention that they have received. This is not a new issue. In fact, it is closely related to statistical thinking and research on analysis of observational data and causal inference. For example, as early as 1968, William G. Cochran considered the use of stratification and subclassification as a tool for removing bias in observational studies. In a now classic example, Cochran examined the relationship between mortality and smoking using data from a large medical database (Cochran, 1968). The first row of Table 2-1 shows that cigarette smoking is unrelated to mortality, but pipe smoking appears to be quite lethal. The result of this early data-mining exercise could have easily misled researchers for some time at the

TABLE 2-1 Smoking and Mortality

	Mortality (%) per 1,000 Person-Years		
Stratification or subclassification	Nonsmokers	Cigarette Smokers	Pipe and Cigar Smokers
One (all ages in database)	13.5	13.5	17.4
Two	13.5	16.4	14.9
Three	13.5	17.7	14.2
Ten	13.5	21.2	13.7

SOURCE: Cochran (1968).

early stages of scientific discovery. It turns out that, at least at the time that these data were collected, pipe smokers were on average much older than cigarette smokers, hence the false association with an increased rate of mortality in the non-stratified group. Cochran (1968) illustrated the effect that stratification (i.e., by age) has on the direction and ultimate interpretation of the results, revealing the association between cigarette smoking and mortality (Table 2-1).

It might be argued that a good data analyst would never have made this mistake because such an analyst would have tested for relevant interactions with important variables such as age. However, the simple statistical solution to this problem can also be misleading in an analysis of observational data. For example, nothing in the statistical output alerts the analyst to a potential nonoverlap in the marginal distributions. An investigator may be comparing 70-year-old smokers with 40-year-old nonsmokers, whereas traditional statistical approaches assume that the groups have the same covariate distributions and the statistical analyses are often limited to linear adjustments and extrapolation. Cochran illustrated that some statistical approaches (e.g., stratification or subclassification) produced more robust solutions when they were applied to naturalistic data than when they were applied to other types of data. Rosenbaum and Rubin (1983) extended the notion of subclassification to the multivariate case (i.e., more than one stratification variable) by introducing the propensity score. Propensity score matching allows the matching of cases and controls in terms of their propensities or probabilities of receiving the intervention on the basis of a number of potentially confounding variables. The result is a matched set of cases and controls that are, in terms of probability, equally likely to have received the treatment. The limitation is that the results from such a comparison will be less generalizable than the results of a randomized study, in which each individual in the total sample has the same likelihood of being a case or a control.

In randomized experiments, ignoring important covariates increases the standard errors of the estimates. By contrast, in observational studies bias can result and the standard errors can be underestimated, leading to an opportunity for a chance association and potentially misleading results. Such problems become more complex as the number of potential outcome variables increase beyond one.

Masking (Blinding)

Investigators in clinical trials use the method of masking (or blinding), in which neither the participant nor the physician, investigator, or evaluator knows who is assigned to the placebo or control group and who will receive the experimental intervention. The purpose of masking is to minimize the occurrences of conscious and unconscious biases in the conduct of a clinical trial and in the interpretation of its results (Pocock, 1984). The knowledge of whether a participant is receiving the intervention under study or is in the control group may have an effect on several aspects of a study, including the recruitment and allocation of participants, their subsequent care, the attitudes of the study participants toward the interventions, the assessment of outcomes, the handling of withdrawals, and the exclusion of data from analysis. The essential aim of masking is to prevent identification of the interventions that individuals are receiving until all opportunities for biases have passed (Pocock, 1984). Many randomized trials that have not used appropriate levels of masking show larger treatment effects than blinded studies (Day and Altman, 2000).

In a *double-blind trial*, neither the participants nor the research or medical staff responsible for the management or clinical evaluation of the individuals knows who is receiving the experimental intervention and who is in the control group. To achieve this, the interventions being compared during the trial must be disguised so that they cannot be distinguished in any way (e.g., by formulation, appearance, or taste) by the research participants or the investigators. Double-blind trials are thought to produce more objective results, because the expectations of the investigators and participants about the experimental intervention do not affect the outcome of the trial.

Although a double-blind study is ideal for the minimization of bias in clinical trials, use of such a study design may not always be feasible. The interventions may be so different that it is not possible to disguise one from the other, for example, surgery versus drug therapy. If sham surgery would be necessary to maintain blinding, ethical problems associated with the use of sham surgery may proscribe the use of a double-blind design. Two drugs may have different forms (e.g., an intravenously administered form versus a tablet form) that cannot be changed without changing the properties of the drugs. One way to design a double-blind trial in this instance is to use a double-dummy technique (e.g., the use of two placebos to disguise which drug the participants are receiving).

An alternative design when a double-blind trial is not feasible is the *single-blind trial.* In a single blind trial the investigators and their colleagues are aware of the intervention but the research participant is not. When blinding is not feasible, an *open-label trial,* in which the identity of the intervention is known to both the investigator and the participants, is used. One way to reduce bias in single blind and open-label trials is for those who conduct all clinical assessments to remain blinded to the assignment of interventions. In single-blind or open-label trials, it is important to place extra emphasis on the minimization of the various known sources of bias as much as possible.

Randomization

Randomization is the process of assigning participants to intervention regimens by using a mechanism of allocation by chance. Random allocation for the comparison of different interventions has been a mainstay of experimental designs since the pioneering work of Ronald A. Fisher. Fisher conducted randomized experiments in agriculture in which the experimental units were plots of land to which various crops and fertilizers were assigned in a random arrangement (Fisher, 1935). Randomization guards against the use of judgment or systematic arrangements that would lead to biased results. Randomization introduces a deliberate element of chance into the assignment of interventions to participants and therefore is intended to provide a sound statistical basis for the evaluation of the effects of the intervention (Pocock, 1984). In clinical research, randomization protects against selection bias in treatment assignment and minimizes the differences among groups by optimizing the likelihood of equally distributing people with particular characteristics to the intervention and control arms of a trial. In randomized experiments, ignoring important covariates, which can lead to differences between the groups, simply increases the standard errors; however, in observational studies, bias can result and the standard errors are underestimated.

There are several different randomization methods (Friedman, Furberg, and DeMets, 1996). Some of these procedures are designed to ensure balance among intervention groups with respect to important prognostic factors, and thus, the probability of assignment to a particular intervention may change over the course of the trial. Thus, randomization does not always imply that an individual participant has a 50 percent chance of being assigned to a particular intervention.

Clinical trials can use either *randomized controls* or *nonrandomized controls*. In a trial with nonrandomized controls, the choice of intervention group and control group is decided deliberately. For example, patients with a specific disease characteristic are assigned to the experimental intervention, whereas those with another disease characteristic are assigned to the control arm. On scientific grounds it is easy to conclude that the use of a randomized control group is always preferred. The consensus view among clinical investigators is that, in general, the use of nonrandomized controls can result in biased and unreliable results (Pocock, 1984). Randomization in combination with masking helps to avoid possible bias in the selection of participants, their assignment to an intervention or control, and the analysis of their response to the intervention.

Outcomes

The health outcomes assessed are pivotal for both the scientific and substantive credibilities of all trials—and are even more pivotal for small trials. The selection of outcomes should meet the guidelines for validity (Tugwell and Bombardier, 1982). In psychology, the concepts of validity and reliability have been developed with the view that measurement is mainly done to discriminate between states and to prognosticate from a single measurement. For example, an intelligence test can be administered to children at the end of their primary school years to suggest the needed level of secondary education. In clinical trials, however, measurement of change (e.g., to monitor the effect of treatment) is the objective. Thus, the concept of responsiveness or sensitivity to change becomes important, but its nomenclature and methodology have not been well developed. In the selection of outcome measures, validity is not the only issue—feasibility also determines which of the valid outcome measures can actually be applied. The most important criteria for selecting an endpoint include truth, discrimination and feasibility (Boers, Brooks, Strand, et al., 1998, 1999).

- *Truth.* Truth captures issues of fact, content, construct, and criterion validity. For example, is the measure truthful, does it measure what is intended? Is the result unbiased and relevant?
- *Discrimination.* Discrimination captures issues of reliability and responsiveness or sensitivity to change. For example, does the measure discriminate between situations of interest? The situations can be states at one time (for classification or prognosis) or states at different times (to measure change).
- *Feasibility.* Feasibility captures an essential element in the selection of measures, one that may be decisive in determining a measure's success. For example, can the measure be applied easily, given constraints of time, money, and interpretability?

Subject Populations

Any clinical trial design requires precision in the process by which participants are determined to be eligible for inclusion. The objective is to ensure that participants in a clinical trial are representative of some future class of patients or individuals to whom the trial's findings might be applied (Pocock, 1984). In the early phases of clinical trial development, research participants are often selected from a small subgroup of the population in which the intervention might eventually be used. This is done to maximize the chance of observing the specific clinical effects of interest. In these early stages it is sometimes necessary to compromise and study a somewhat less representative group (Pocock, 1984). Similarly, preliminary data collected from one population (e.g., from studies of bone mineral density loss in ground-based study participants) may not be generalizable to a particular target population of interest (astronauts).

Sample Size and Statistical Power

Numerous methods and statistical models, often called "power calculations," have been developed to calculate sample sizes (Kraemer and Thiemann, 1987) (see also Chapter 3). A standard approach asks five questions:

1. What is the main purpose of the trial?
2. What is the principal method of assessing patient outcomes?
3. How will the data be analyzed to detect treatment differences?
4. What results does one anticipate with standard treatment?

5. How small a treatment difference is it important to detect, and with what degree of certainty should that treatment difference be demonstrated?

Statistical methods can then be developed around qualitative or quantitative outcomes. A critical aspect of trial design is to first make use of statistical methods to determine the population size needed to determine the feasibility of the clinical trial. The number of participants in a clinical trial should always be large enough to provide a sufficiently precise answer to the question posed, but it should also be the minimum necessary to achieve this aim.

A trial with only a small number of participants carries a considerable risk of failing to demonstrate a treatment difference when one is really present (Type II error) (see the Glossary for explanations of Type I and Type II errors). In general, small studies are more prone to variability and thus are likely to be able to detect only large intervention effects with adequate statistical power.

Components of Variance

Variance is a measure of the dispersion or variation of data within a population distribution. In the example of the effects of microgravity on bone mineral density loss during space travel (see Box 1-2), there is a tendency to assume that the astronaut is the unit of analysis and hence to focus on components of variance across astronauts. However, given that astronauts comprise a small group of individuals and do not represent a larger population, there is a great likelihood that the data distribution will be less of a Gaussian (or a "normal") distribution. In this case, it becomes important to consider the other components of variance in addition to the among-person variance.

In a study of bone mineral density loss among astronauts, the components of variance may include:

1. variation in bone mineral density across time for a single astronaut on Earth or in microgravity;
2. differences in bone mineral density for that astronaut on Earth and after a fixed period of time in microgravity; and
3. differences in bone mineral density among astronauts both on Earth and in microgravity.

The goal would be to characterize changes for an individual astronaut or a small group of astronauts, even though they do not perfectly represent a large population. It is reasonable to focus on true trends for a particular astronaut over time, which requires careful repeated measurements over time and which makes relevant the component of variance within a person rather than the component of variance among persons.

Significance Tests

Significance tests (e.g., chi-square and *t* tests) are used to determine the chances of finding a treatment difference as large as the effect observed by chance alone; that is, how strong is the evidence for a genuine superiority of one intervention over another (see also Chapter 3). However, statistical significance is not the same as clinical or societal significance. Clinical or societal significance (relevance) must be assessed in terms of whether the magnitude of the observed effect is meaningful in the context of established clinical practice or public health. An increase of risk from 1 in 10 to 2 in 10 has a clinical implication different from that of an increase of 1 in 10,000 to 2 in 10,000, even though the risk has doubled in each case.

In hypothesis testing, the null hypothesis and one's confidence in either its validation or refute are the issue:

> The basic overall principle is that the researcher's theory is considered false until demonstrated beyond reasonable doubt to be true... This is expressed as an assumption that the *null hypothesis*, the contradiction of the researcher's theory, is true... What is considered a "reasonable" doubt is called the *significance level*. By convention in scientific research, a "reasonable" level of remaining doubt is one below either 5% or 1%. A statistical test defines a rule that, when applied to the data, determines whether the null hypothesis can be rejected... Both the significance level and the power of the test are derived by calculating with what probability a positive verdict would be obtained (the null hypothesis rejected) if the same trial were run over and over again (Kraemer and Thiemann, 1987, pp. 22–23).

A clinical trial is often formulated as a hypothesis as to whether an experimental therapy is effective. However, confidence intervals may provide a better indication of the level of uncertainty. In the clinical trial setting, the hypothesis test is natural, because the goal is to determine whether an experimental therapy should be used. In clinical trials, confidence intervals are used in the same manner as hypothesis tests. Thus, if the interval includes the null hypothesis, one concludes that the experimental therapy has not proved to be more effective than the control.

To obtain the significance level, hypothetical repeats of trials are done when the null hypothesis is taken to be true. To obtain power, repeat tests are done when the alternative hypothesis is correct. To compute power, the researcher must have developed from preliminary data a *critical-effect size*, that is, a measure of how strong the theory must minimally be to be important to the individual being offered the therapy or important to society (Kraemer and Thiemann, 1987, p. 24). Changing designs or measures used or choosing one valid test over another changes the definition of effect size. Moreover, the critical-effect size is individual- or population-specific as well as measurement-specific (Kraemer and Thiemann, 1987).

TRADITIONAL CLINICAL TRIAL DESIGNS

Modern clinical trials go back more than 40 years, and a wide variety of clinical trial designs have been developed and adapted over the past 25 years. To the extent possible, each of these designs uses the concepts of control and randomization to make comparisons among groups (Box 2-2). Some of these designs, which are generally used in larger studies, can also be adapted for use in some small studies. For example, crossover designs can be used in small clinical studies and can be used in within-subject trials. Each is described below.

Parallel-Group Design

The most common clinical trial design is the *parallel-group design*, in which participants are randomized to one of two or more arms (Pocock, 1984). These arms include the new intervention under investigation and one or more control arms, such as a placebo control or an active control. The randomized parallel-group design is typically used to evaluate differences in

BOX 2-2
Traditional Designs for Clinical Trials

Parallel-group design
Crossover design
Factorial design
Add-on design
Randomized withdrawal design
Early-escape design

the effects of different interventions across time. Trials that use the parallel-group design are often double blinded. Because of the improved ability to control for bias through randomization and blinding, the analysis of such trials and the interpretation of their results are generally straightforward.

Crossover Design

The *crossover design* compares two or more interventions by randomly assigning each participant to receive the interventions being tested in a different sequence. Once one intervention is completed, participants are switched to another intervention. For example, in a two-by-two crossover design, each participant randomly receives one drug for one period of time and then another drug for a second period of time, with the administration of each drug separated by a washout period (i.e., a period of time during which the first drug is cleared from the body before the second drug is administered). With this type of study, each participant serves as his or her own control. There are several advantages to this trial design, including a reduction in the number of participants required to achieve a statistically significant result and the ability to control for patient specific effects. This design can also be useful for studying a patient's response to short periods of therapy, particularly for chronic conditions in which the initial evaluation of treatment efficacy is concerned with the measurement of short-term relief of symptoms (Pocock, 1984).

A criticism of this design is that the effects of one intervention may carry over into the period when the next intervention is given. Crossover studies cannot be done if the effects of the interventions are irreversible (e.g., gene therapy or surgery) or the disease progression is not stable over time (e.g., advanced cancer). Additional problems with crossover studies occur if participants withdraw from the study before they receive both interventions or the outcomes are affected by the order in which the interventions are administered (Senn, 1993).

Crossover designs are occasionally used in psychological studies because of the opportunity to use each patient at least twice and because of the probability that the component of the variance within individual patients is smaller than between patients (Matthews, 1995).

Factorial Design

In a *factorial design*, two or more treatments are evaluated simultaneously with the same participant population through the use of various combinations of the treatments. For example, in a two-by-two factorial design, participants are randomly allocated to one of the four possible combinations of two treatments, treatments A and B: treatment A alone, treatment B alone, both treatments A and B, or neither treatment A nor treatment B. The usual intention of using this design is to make efficient use of clinical trial participants by evaluating the efficacies of the two treatments with the same number of participants that would be required to evaluate the efficacy of either one alone. The success of this approach depends on the absence of any relevant interaction between treatments A and B so that the effect of treatment A is virtually identical whether or not treatment B is administered. This design can also be used to test the interaction of treatments A and B, but then, the advantages of efficiency no longer apply because much larger trials are necessary to detect a clinically relevant interaction.

The factorial design can also be used to establish the dose-response characteristics of a combination product, for example, one that combines treatments C and D. Different doses of treatment C are selected, usually including a dose of zero (placebo), and similar doses of treatment D are also chosen. Participants in each arm of the trial receive a different combination of doses of treatments C and D. The resulting estimate of the response may then be used to help to identify an appropriate combination of doses of treatments C and D for clinical use.

Add-on Design

In an *add-on design*, a placebo-controlled trial of an experimental intervention is tested with people already receiving an established, effective treatment. Thus, all participants receive the established, effective treatment. The add-on design is especially useful for the testing of experimental interventions that have a mechanism of action different from that of the established, effective treatment. Experimental interventions for patients with acute myocardial infarctions and, increasingly, patients with rheumatoid arthritis, for example, are often tested in studies with this design. The add-on design is the only one that can be used in long-term studies of treatments for heart failure since standard therapy is lifesaving and cannot be denied (Temple, 1996). However, the add-on design is most useful for the testing of experimental interventions that have mechanisms of action different from that of the established, effective treatment.

Randomized Withdrawal Design

In a *randomized withdrawal design*, individuals who respond positively to an experimental intervention are randomized to continue receiving that intervention or to receive a placebo. This trial design minimizes the amount of time that individuals receive a placebo (Temple, 1996). During the trial, the return of symptoms or the ability to continue participation in the trial are study endpoints (Temple, 1996). The advantages of this study design are that individuals receiving the experimental intervention continue to do so only if they respond, whereas individuals receiving the placebo do so only until their symptoms return. Disadvantages include carryover effects, difficulties assessing whether the underlying disease process is still active, and long lag times to adverse events if the disease is in remission. This design is more appropriate in phase I and II trials involving healthy volunteers because it is less likely that effective treatments are being withdrawn from those who need it. In some studies, however, measurement of the placebo effect is essential (e.g., studies of drugs for the treatment of depression), and such studies might require the use of a randomized withdrawal design. In those cases, voluntary, informed consent is essential, as is the provision of care during the withdrawal period.

Early-Escape Design

The *early-escape design* is another way to minimize an individual's duration of exposure to a placebo. In the early-escape design, participants are removed from the study if symptoms reach a defined level or they fail to respond to a defined extent. The failure rate can then be used as the measure of efficacy. Thus, in a study with an early-escape design, participants are only briefly exposed to ineffective interventions (Temple, 1996).

Multicenter Trials

Multicenter trials, although not a traditional design, provide an efficient way of establishing the efficacy of a new intervention; however, certain caveats must be noted. Sometimes multicenter trials provide the only means of accruing a sample of sufficient size within a reasonable time frame. Another advantage of multicenter trials is that they provide a better basis for the subsequent generalization of findings because the participants are recruited from a wider population and the treatment is administered in a broader range of clinical settings. In this sense, the environment in which a multicenter trial is conducted might more truly represent the environment for future uses of the test intervention. On the other hand, multicenter trials may require the use of multiple standards and quality control.

SPECIAL DESIGN ISSUES FOR SMALL TRIALS

A number of trial designs especially lend themselves to studies with small numbers of participants, including single subject (*n*-of-1) designs, sequential designs, decision analysis-based designs, ranking and selection designs, adaptive designs, and risk-based allocation designs (Box 2-3).

Conducting Randomized Trials with Individual Patients

Clinicians are often faced with treatment decisions when they cannot rely on the results of an RCT because the results do not apply to that patient or a relevant trial might not yet have been done. In this case, the clinician might opt for a "trial of therapy"; that is, the clinician might administer more than one treatment to a patient to assess the effects (Guyatt, Sackett, Adachi, et al., 1988). Trials with this type of design (referred to as a trial with an *n*-of-1 design) have a long tradition in the behavioral sciences and have more recently been used in clinical medicine (Johannessen, 1991). Trials with such designs can improve the certainty of a treatment decision for a single patient; a series of trials with such designs may permit more general inferences to be drawn about a specific treatment approach (Johannessen, 1991). They also become useful when a population is believed to be heterogeneous. The central premise of trials with such designs is that the patient (e.g., an astronaut) serves as his or her own control.

The factors that can mislead physicians conducting conventional therapeutic trials—the placebo effect, the natural history of the illness, and ex-

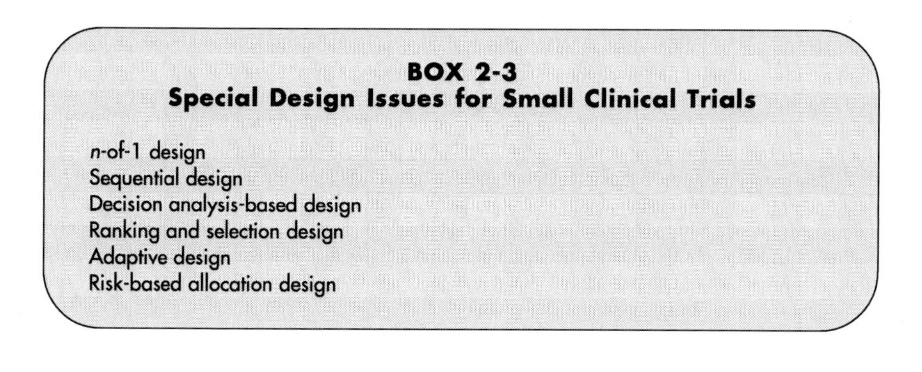
BOX 2-3
Special Design Issues for Small Clinical Trials

n-of-1 design
Sequential design
Decision analysis-based design
Ranking and selection design
Adaptive design
Risk-based allocation design

pectations about the treatment effect—can be avoided in trials of therapy with *n*-of 1-designs by safeguards that permit the natural, untreated course of the disorder to be observed and by keeping the patient and the clinician blind to the timing of active treatment.

Guyatt and colleagues (1988) describe one method of conducting an RCT with an *n*-of-1 design:

- A clinician and a patient agree to test a therapy (the "experimental therapy") for its ability to reduce or control the symptoms, signs, or other manifestations (the "treatment targets") of the patient's ailment.
- The patient then undergoes treatment for a pair of periods; during one period of each pair the experimental therapy is applied, and during the other period either an alternative treatment or a placebo is applied. The order of the two periods within each pair is randomized by a method that ensures that each period has an equal chance of applying the experimental or the alternative therapy.
- Whenever possible both the clinician and the patient are blind to the treatment being given during either period.
- The treatment targets are monitored (often through the use of a patient diary) to document the effect of the treatment being applied.
- Pairs of treatment periods are replicated until the clinician and the patient are convinced that the experimental therapy is effective, is harmful, or has no effect on the treatment targets.

RCTs with *n*-of 1 designs may be indicated if an RCT has shown that some patients are unresponsive to treatment, if there is doubt about whether a treatment is really providing a benefit to a particular patient; when the patient insists on taking a treatment that the clinician thinks is useless or potentially harmful, when a patient is experiencing symptoms suspected to be medication side effects but neither the patient nor the clinician is certain, and when neither the clinician nor the patient is confident of the optimal dose of a medication or replacement therapy (Edgington, 1996). In addition, RCTs with *n*-of-1 designs are most useful for the study of treatments for chronic conditions for which maintenance therapy is likely to be continued for long periods of time and if the treatment effect occurs soon after the initiation of treatment and ceases soon after the withdrawal of treatment. Trials with *n*-of 1 designs are also attractive for the study of vaguely defined or heterogeneous conditions (Table 2-2). For patients with these conditions, studies with *n*-of-1 designs may generate new hypotheses for the design of

TABLE 2-2 Considerations in Performing a Trial with an *n*-of-1 Design

Is the condition chronic?
Is the condition stable over time?
Is there a carryover effect?
Is there a period effect?
Do the effects of the treatments have a rapid onset or a rapid cessation?
Are good measures available for the evaluation of the response?
Is a blinded trial feasible?
Is treatment effectiveness uncertain for the individual?
Is long-term therapy being considered?
Is the optimal dose known?
Is treatment timing feasible?
Is the patient interested in participating in a trial with an *n*-of-1 design?
Is the trial feasible in the clinician's practice?
Is the trial ethical?

SOURCE: Zucker (2000).

subsequent conventional group trials and can bridge the gap between research and clinical practice (Johannessen, 1991).

One concern about trials with *n*-of-1 designs is whether clinically relevant targets of treatment can be measured. Outcome measures often extend beyond a set of physical signs (e.g., the rigidity and tremor of parkinsonism), laboratory tests (e.g., measurement of blood glucose levels), or a measure of patient performance (e.g., score on a 6-minute walking test). Thus, in most situations it is preferable to directly measure a patient's symptoms, well being, or quality of life. The measurement of a patient's symptoms may also include the side effects of treatment (Guyatt, Sackett, Adachi, et al., 1988).

One of the advantages to not specifying the number of pairs of treatment periods in advance is that the trial can be stopped at any time. If, on the other hand, one wishes to conduct a standard statistical analysis of data (e.g., a frequentist or a Bayesian analysis), the analysis will be strengthened considerably if the number of pairs is specified in advance. Regardless of whether the number of treatment periods is specified in advance, it is advisable to have at least two pairs of treatment periods before breaking the trial (Guyatt, 1986). Conclusions drawn after a single pair of treatments are likely to be either false positive (that the treatment is effective when it is not) or false negative (that the treatment is not effective when it is). Moreover, a positive effect of treatment in one patient is not a reliable predictor of the responses in future patients.

A preliminary treatment period with active therapy, during which both the clinician and the patient know that active therapy is being received, could save time. If there is no evidence of a response during such an open trial or if intolerable side effects occur, an RCT with an *n*-of-1 design may be meaningless or impossible. An open preliminary treatment period may also be used to determine the optimal dose of the medication to be used in the trial.

If requirements similar to those required for conventional group trials—strict entry criteria, uniform treatment procedures, consensus scales for outcome measures, and acceptable statistical tests—are applied to a series of trials with *n*-of-1 designs, conclusions may be generalizable to the target population (Johannessen, 1991; Zucker, Schmid, McIntosh, et al., 1997). This has the advantage that the patients are exposed to placebo only for as long as is needed to get an answer both for the patients and for the main population database.

A repeated-measures design is likely to be very useful in small studies. The extreme of a small repeated-measures design is the study with an *n*-of-1 design. At the design phase of a study with a repeated-measures design, the correlation structure of the measures is an important parameter. One would need to explore the feasibility (i.e., the statistical power) of the study under several different assumptions about the correlation structure.

Sequential Designs

In a study with a sequential design, participants are sequentially enrolled in the study and are assigned a treatment (assignment is usually at random). The investigator then changes the probabilities that participants will be assigned to any particular treatment on the basis of as they become available. The object is to improve the efficiency, safety, or efficacy of the experiment as it is in progress by changing the rules by which one determines how participants are allocated to the various treatments.

Strategies for sequential dose-response designs include up-and-down methods, stochastic approximation methods, maximum-likelihood methods, and Bayesian methods. Recently, attention has been focused on the continual reassessment methods which is a Bayesian sequential design (Durham, Flournoy, and Rosenberger, 1997). Random-walk rules are particularly attractive for use in the design of dose-response studies for several reasons: exact finite and asymptotic distribution theory is completely worked out, which allows the experimenter to choose design parameters for the most ethical allocation scheme; specific designs can be chosen that allow the chosen design points to be distributed unimodally around a quantile of interest; the designs are very simple to implement; and the designs operate on a finite lattice of dosages (Durham, Flournoy, and Rosenberger, 1997). Random-walk rules identify a class of rules for which the sample paths form random walks. Thus, if there is a fixed probability of transitioning from state A to state B and another fixed probability of transitioning from state B to state A in a two-state process (a Markov chain), then sequences of states such as A, B, B, A, B,... are random walks. A rule such as "stop the first time that the total number of A's or B's reaches a prespecified number" would be called a random-walk rule.

One example of sequential design is called the "up-and-down design" (Dixon and Mood, 1948), in which the choices of experimental treatment either go up one level (dose), down one level (dose), or stay unchanged. The design allocates treatments to pairs of participants in a way that causes the treatment distribution to cluster around the treatment with a maximum probability of success (Dixon and Mood, 1948; Kpamegan and Flournoy, 2001). An up-and-down design has some advantages in clinical trials, in that it allows more conservative movement across a range of treatments. To optimize an up-and-down design, one treats individuals in pairs, with one receiving the lower-dose treatment and the other receiving the higher-dose treatment. If the lower-dose treatment results in a treatment failure and the higher-dose treatment results in a treatment success, the doses of the treatment are increased for the next pair. Conversely, if the patient with the lower-dose treatment has a treatment success and the patient with the higher-dose treatment has a treatment failure, then the doses of the treatment are decreased for the next pair. In this simple model, if there are two treatment successes or two treatment failures, the study is stopped. This design allows early estimations of the effective dosage range to be obtained before investigators proceed with large-scale randomized trials (Flournoy, in press).

Sequential group designs are useful for the monitoring and accumulation of study data, while they preserve the Type I error probability at a desired significance level, despite the repeated application of significance tests (Kim and DeMets, 1992). Parallel-groups are studied until a clear benefit is seen or it is determined that no difference in treatments exists (Lai, Levin, Robbins, et al., 1980; Whitehead, 1999). The sequential group design allows results to be monitored at specific time intervals throughout the trial so that the trial may be stopped early if there is clear evidence of efficacy. Safety monitoring can also be done, and trials can be stopped early if unacceptable adverse effects occur or if it is determined that the chance of showing a clinically valuable benefit is futile. Because there is a need in all clinical trials—as dictated by ethical requirements—to assess results throughout the course of the trial, there is a potential that the blind will be broken, depending on how the results are assessed and by whom.

The disadvantage of this approach is that in most trials patients are heterogeneous with respect to the important prognostic factors, and these methods do not protect against the introduction of bias as a result of changes in the types of patients entering into a clinical trial over time. Moreover, for patients with chronic diseases, responses are usually delayed so long that the advantages of this approach are often lost.

Decision Analysis-Based Design

Decision analysis (Pauker, 2000) can be informative in the experimental design process. Modeling of a clinical situation a priori allows testing of variables, which allows determination of the potential impact of each variable on the decision. Framing the question starts the decision analysis-based design process.

One explicitly considers both decision (e.g., intervention A or intervention B) and probabilistic events (e.g., side effect versus no side effect). A utility is assigned to each outcome. Utilities have numeric values, usually between 0 and 1, that reflect the desirability of an outcome; that is, they incorporate the weighting of the severity or importance of the possible adverse outcomes as well as the weighting of the severity or importance of the beneficial outcomes (Drummond, O'Brien, Stoddart, et al., 1997). Decision analysis combines the probability of each outcome with the utility to calculate an expected utility for each decision.

During the planning phase for a study, decision analysis is used to structure the question. One obtains (either from data or from expert opinion) best estimates for each probability and utility. One then varies potential important values (either probability or utility) over a likely range. This process, known as "sensitivity analysis," allows the design group to determine if the decision is sensitive to that value. Thus, decision analysis can direct small trials to focus on these important variables. The integrity of an analysis depends both on the values and on the model's structure. One should make both values and structure available for evaluation. One can use the process of varying the value assumptions (known as sensitivity analysis) to determine if a value's precision would change one's decision. It is important to recognize, however, that decision analysis is dependent on the assumptions made about parameter values and model structure. Reviews of decision analyses should include careful critique of the model structure. (See Chapter 3 for a further discussion and an example of decision analysis.)

Ranking and Selection Design

Selection problems pervade the conduct of clinical trials. Statisticians can provide rational procedures for selection of the best of several alternatives. The *formulation* of the goal for the statistical significance of a trial influences sample size in a substantial way. The hypothesis test has been the predominant formulation used in the design of large-scale, randomized trials, but other paradigms deserve careful consideration, especially in situations with small sample sizes. One such paradigm is ranking and selection. Ranking and selection procedures are statistical techniques for comparison of the parameters for multiple study (k) populations under the assumption that these parameters are not all the same (Gibbons, Olkin, and Sobel, 1979). The methods, known generally as *ranking and selection procedures*, include techniques appropriate for the achievement of many different goals, although a careful formulation of the corresponding problem is needed for each goal. Suppose there are k populations and that each population is characterized by a parameter. For example, the k populations are normally distributed with different means and a common variance. In this context, populations for which mean values are large are preferable to populations for which mean values are small. For any given set of k populations, some of the goals that can be accomplished by these methods are

1. selection of the one best population;
2. selection of a random number of populations such that all populations better than a control population or a standard are included in the selected subset;
3. selection of the t best populations for $t \geq 2$ (a) in an ordered manner or (b) in an unordered manner;
4. selection of a random number of populations, say r, which includes the t best populations;
5. selection of a fixed number of populations, say r, which includes the t best populations;
6. ordering of all the k populations from best to worst (or vice versa); or
7. ordering of a fixed-size subset of the populations from best to worst (or vice versa) (Gibbons, Olkin, and Sobel, 1979).

Ranking and selection procedures are particularly appropriate for answering questions such as the following (Gibbons, Olkin, and Sobel, 1979):

- Which one of λ different drugs produces the best response?
- Which subgroup of the λ drugs produces a better response than a placebo?
- Which two of α types of advertising media reach the largest proportion of potential buyers of a particular product?
- Which one of β different learning techniques produces the best comprehension?

Instead of formulating the goal of a trial as the definitive rejection of a null hypothesis when it is false (with a high degree of statistical power) while limiting its rejection when it is true (at a given level of a Type I error rate) in planning a selection trial a clinician might reason as explained in Box 2-4.

A related goal is to rank three or more treatments in order of preference. Methods for ranking and selection lend themselves naturally to sequentialization. Sequential selection procedures can further reduce the sample size required to select the best of two or more treatments (Levin and Robbins, 1981). One of the ways in which ranking and selection methods can be of help in a process is by ruling out poor competitors. Suppose that investigators must choose the best of five interventions. With small sample sizes the investigators may not be able to choose the best but might be able

BOX 2-4
Example of a Selection Trial

Over the course of the coming year, a clinician will have *N* patients to treat with disease D. The clinician can treat these patients with therapy A or therapy B, but it is unclear which therapy is better. One thing is clear, however: the clinician must treat all patients with one or the other therapy and is willing to conduct a trial in which the goal is, ideally, to select the truly superior treatment. If the two treatments are in truth equally effective (with other factors such as cost and side effects being equal), the clinician should be indifferent to which therapy is selected. If one treatment is sufficiently better than the other, however, the clinician wants a high degree of probability that he or she will select the superior treatment.

In other words, the traditional hypothesis test is used for the formulation of confirmatory trials, but a selection trial identifies for further use a therapy that is sufficiently superior with a guaranteed high degree of probability. On the other hand, if the therapies are essentially equivalent, the goal is to be able to select either therapy. Because it is possible to view such selection trials as equivalent to classical hypothesis testing with a Type I error rate of 0.5 (rather than a Type I error rate of 0.05), it can be seen that selection trials generally require much smaller sample sizes than those required for the usual confirmatory trial. Note that this is not a way of cheating but is an explicit decision to acknowledge the importance of the selection paradigm over the definitive or confirmatory hypothesis test paradigm.

to assert that the best is among a group of three of the interventions, although they are not sure which one is the best. Subsequent studies can then focus on choosing the best of the three interventions.

A key criterion in selection trials is the probability of selection of the "correct" treatment. Even more intriguing criteria have been proposed for the selection of a superior treatment. In a review of the second edition of Peter Armitage's book *Sequential Medical Trials*, Frank Anscombe introduced what has been called the "ethical cost" function, which considers the number of inferior treatments and the severity of such treatments errors (Lai, Levin, Robbins, et al., 1980).

Consider again the finite patient horizon of N patients to be treated over the course of a given time period. Suppose n pairs of patients (for a total of $2n$ patients) are to be considered in the trial phase, with treatment A or treatment B randomly allocated within pairs. After the trial phase, the remaining $N - 2n$ patients will all be given the apparently superior treatment identified in the trialphase. The ethical cost function is the total number of patients given the truly inferior treatment multiplied by the magnitude of the treatment efficacy difference. If (AD) denotes the absolute difference in average endpoint levels between the two treatments, then the ethical cost is $(AD)n$ if the truly superior treatment is selected in the trial phase and $(AD)(N - n)$ if the truly superior treatment is not selected.

It is simple to implement a sequential version of the trial phase; it also has the virtue of achieving a substantially lower average ethical cost than that which can be achieved with a fixed sample size in the trial phase. A surprising feature of a large class of reasonable sequential stopping rules for the trial phase is that they can reduce the average ethical cost for a fixed sample size, even when the ethical cost is optimized for a given value of (AD). For example, one such rule will reach a decision in the trial phase in which n is no more than one-sixth of N. The main point for consideration in small trials, however, is that it may not be obvious how one rationalizes the trade-off between the number of patients put at risk in the trial and an ultimately arbitrary Type I error rate in a conventional trial. On the other hand, it may be much more desirable to design a selection trial with an ethical cost function that directly incorporates the number of patients given inferior treatment.

Adaptive Design

Adaptive designs have been suggested as a way to overcome the ethical dilemmas that arise when the early results from an RCT clearly begin to favor one intervention over another. An adaptive design seeks to skew assignment probabilities to favor the better-performing treatment in a trial that is under way (Rosenberger, 1996).

Adaptive designs are attractive to mathematicians and statisticians because they impose dependencies that require the full arsenal of techniques and stochastic processes (Rosenberger, 1996). An assortment of adaptive designs has been developed over the past few decades, including a variety of urn models that govern the sampling mechanism. Adaptive design can be associated with complex analytical problems. If the sample size is small enough, an exact analysis by exhaustive enumeration of all sample paths is one way to provide an answer. If the sample size is larger but still not large, a Monte Carlo simulation can provide an accurate analysis. If the sample size is large, then standard likelihood-based methods can be used. An example of an adaptive design is described in Box 2-5.

A major advantage of adaptive design is that over time more patients will be assigned to the more successful treatment. Stopping rules and data analysis for these types of designs are complicated (Hoel, Sobel, and Weiss, 1975), and more research is needed in this area. As with sequential designs, the disadvantage of adaptive designs is that in most trials, patients are heterogeneous with respect to the important prognostic factors, and these methods do not protect against bias introduced by changes in the types of patients entering into a trial over time. Morever, for patients with chronic diseases, responses are usually delayed so long that the advantages of this approach are often lost. Also, multiple endpoints are usually of interest, and therefore, the entire allocation process should not be based on a single response. Play-the-winner rules can be useful in certain specialized medical situations in which ethical challenges are strong and one can be reasonably certain that time trends and patient heterogeneity are unimportant. These

BOX 2-5
Play-the-Winner Rule as an Example of Adaptive Design

A simple version of a randomized version of the play-the-winner rule follows. An urn contains two balls; one is labeled A and the other is labeled B. When a patient is available for treatment assignment, a ball is drawn at random and replaced. If the ball is type A, the patient is assigned to treatment A; if it is type B, the patient is assigned to treatment B. When the results for a patient are available, the contents of the urn are changed according to the following rule: if the result was a success, an additional ball labeled with the successful treatment is added to the urn. If the result is a failure, a ball with the opposite label is added to the urn (Zelen, 1969).

rules can be especially beneficial when response times are short compared with the times between patient entries into a study. An example of this is the development of extracorporeal membrane oxygenation (Truog, 1992; Ware, 1989).

Risk-Based Allocation Design

Risk-based allocation, a nonrandomized design, has a very specific purpose: to allow individuals at higher risk or with greater disease severity to benefit from a potentially superior experimental treatment. Because the design is nonrandomized, its use should be considered only in situations in which an RCT would not be possible.

For example, when a therapy is readily available outside the study protocol or when a treatment has been in use for a long time and is perceived to be efficacious, even though it has never been subjected to a randomized trial, a nonrandomized risk-based allocation approach may be useful. Bone marrow transplantation for the treatment of advanced breast disease is an illustration. A nationwide, multicenter randomized trial was designed to test the efficacy of harvesting bone marrow before aggressive chemotherapy followed by bone marrow transplantation with the patient's own (autologous) bone marrow for women with at least 10 axillary nodes with tumor involvement. The comparison group received the standard therapy at that time which omitted the bone marrow transplantation procedure. Bone marrow transplantation was widely available outside the clinical trial, and women were choosing that therapy in large numbers, drastically slowing patient enrollment in the trial. It took more than 7 years (between 1991 and 1998) to achieve the target sample size of 982 women, whereas more than 15,000 off-protocol bone marrow transplantation procedures were administered during that time period. If only half of the women receiving off-protocol bone marrow transplantation had been enrolled in the trial, the target sample size would have been reached in less than 2 years. The difficulty was that when participants were informed that they faced a 50 percent chance of being randomized to the comparison group, they withheld consent to obtain bone marrow transplantation elsewhere, often just across town. The final result of the trial was that there was no survival benefit to this approach. A risk-based allocation design might have reached the same conclusion much sooner, saving many women from undergoing a very painful, expensive, and, ultimately, questionable surgical procedure.

Other examples of desperately ill patients or their caregivers seeking experimental treatments and refusing to be randomized include patients with

AIDS in the early days of trials of drugs for the treatment of human immunodeficiency virus infection and caregivers of premature infants with extracorporeal membrane oxygenation. Other therapies, such as pulmonary artery (Swan-Ganz) catheter placement, estrogen treatment for Alzheimer's disease, or radical surgery for prostate cancer, have been nearly impossible to test in randomized trials because participants, convinced of their therapeutic benefits, did not want to receive the placebo or the standard therapy. These therapies have been cited in the news media because of the extreme difficulty in recruiting participants into randomized trials of the therapies (Altman, 1996; Brody, 1997; Kolata, 1995, 1997; Kolata and Eichenwald, 1999).

A risk-based allocation design attempts to circumvent these problems by ensuring that all of the sickest patients will receive the experimental treatment. The design is sometimes called an "assured allocation design" (Finkelstein, Levin, and Robins, 1996a, b). It has also been called the "regression-discontinuity design," although that name presupposes a specific statistical analysis that is not always appropriate.

The design has three novel features. First, it requires a quantitative measure of risk, disease severity, or prognosis, which is observed at or before enrollment in the study, together with a prespecified threshold for receiving the experimental therapy. All participants above the threshold receive the experimental (new) treatment, whereas all participants below the threshold receive the standard (old) treatment. The second novel feature of the risk-based design is the goal of the trial: to estimate the difference in average outcome for high-risk individuals who received the new treatment *compared with that for the same individuals if they had received the old treatment.*

Thus, in the bone marrow transplantation example, women eligible for the randomized trial had to have 10 or more nodes of involvement. In a risk-based allocation trial, all of these high-risk women would have been given bone marrow transplantation, whereas women with fewer affected nodes would have been recruited and given the standard therapy. The treatment effect to be estimated in the assured allocation design would be the survival difference for women with at least 10 nodes given bone marrow transplantation compared with that for the same group of women if they had received the standard therapy.

The risk-based allocation creates a biased allocation, and the statistical analysis appropriate for estimation of the treatment effect is not a simple comparison of the mean outcomes for the two groups, as it would be in a randomized trial. One analytical method comes from the theory of general empirical Bayes estimation, originally introduced by Herbert Robbins in the

1950s in a series of landmark papers (Lai and Siegmund, 1985; Robbins, 1956, 1977). Robbins applied this approach first to estimation problems, then to prediction problems, and later to risk-based allocation (Robbins, 1993; Robbins and Zhang, 1988, 1989, 1991). If one gives up randomization (because the trial would be impossible to carry out), one needs another principle to achieve a scientifically valid estimate of treatment effect. Therefore, the third requirement of risk-based design is a model that can be used to predict what outcomes the sicker patients would have had if they had been given the standard treatment. A prototypic example of the appropriate statistical analysis required is shown in Box 2-6.

Thus, there is good rationale for using a risk-based allocation design to compare the outcomes for high-risk patients who receive the new treatment with the predicted outcome for the same patients if they had received the standard therapy. One requires a model for the standard treatment (but only the standard treatment) that relates the average or expected outcome to specific values of the baseline measure of risk used for the allocation. Only the functional form of the model, not specific values of the model parameters, is required. This is because the parameters used in the model will be estimated from the *concurrent control data*, and extrapolated to the high-risk patients. This is an advantage over historical controlled studies. One need not rely on historical estimates of means or proportions of the expected outcome, which are notoriously untrustworthy. All one needs to assume for the risk-based design is that the mathematical form of the model relating outcome to risk is correctly specified throughout the entire range of the risk measure. This is a strong assumption, but with sufficient experience and prior data on the standard treatment, the form of the model can be validated. In the same way that an engineer can build a bridge without being completely agnostic about the laws of gravity and the tensile strength of steel, so progress can be made without randomization if one has a model that predicts the outcomes of a standard treatment. In addition, the validity of the predictive model can always be checked against the concurrent control data in the risk-based trial.

The usual problem of extrapolation beyond the range of data does not arise here for three reasons. First, one assumes that the mathematical form of the model relating outcome to risk is correctly specified throughout the entire range of the risk measure. If one does not know what lies beyond the range of data, then extrapolation is risky. Thus, in this situation one should assume a validated model for standard treatment that covers the whole range of the risk measure, including data for those high-risk patients that form part of the observed data. Estimation of the model parameters from a por-

BOX 2-6
Example of General Empirical Bayes Estimation

Suppose one collects data on the number of traffic accidents that each driver in a population of motorists had during a 1-year baseline period. Most drivers will have no accidents, some will have one, some will have two, and so on. If one focuses on the subgroup of drivers who had no accidents during the baseline period, one can then ask the following question: assuming that traffic conditions and driving habits remain stable, how many accidents in total would the same drivers with no accident in the baseline year be predicted to have in the next year? A model is needed to make a prediction. A reasonable statistical model is that the number of accidents that a single driver has in a 1-year period follows a Poisson distribution, the standard probability law governing the occurrence of rare events. Subject-to-subject variability requires one to assume that the mean value for a parameter according to a Poisson distribution (the number of accidents expected per year) varies from driver to driver: some drivers have very safe driving habits with a small expected number of accidents per year, whereas others have less safe driving habits.

A key feature of a general empirical Bayes analysis is that *no assumption about the distribution of the Poisson mean parameters in the population of drivers needs be made*. In this case, the term "general empirical Bayes" does not mean empirical Bayes generally but, rather, refers to the kind of empirical Bayes method that does not make assumptions about the prior distribution (in contrast to the parametric variety used by Robbins [1956]). Robbins proved that an unbiased and asymptotically optimal predictor of the number of accidents next year by the drivers who had no accidents in the baseline year is *the number of drivers who had exactly one accident in the baseline year*. The proof of this assertion is based only on the assumption of the form of the model for outcomes (Poisson distribution), without any parametric assumption about how the model parameter is distributed among participants in the population. What is amazing—and the reason that this example is presented—is that information about one group of people (the drivers with no accidents) can be consistently and asymptotically optimally predicted on the basis of information about an entirely different group of people (the drivers with one accident), which is characteristic of empirical Bayes methods. There is no question that the two groups are different: even though the groups of drivers with no accidents includes some unsafe drivers who had no accidents by good fortune, the drivers in that group are, nevertheless, safer drivers on average than the drivers in the group with one accident, even though the latter group includes some safe drivers who were unlucky. This illustrates that the complete homogeneity and comparability of two groups so avidly sought after in randomized comparisons is actually not necessary to make valid comparisons, given adequate model assumptions and an appropriate (not naïve) statistical analysis.

Finally, one can observe the number of accidents next year among those with no accidents in the baseline year and compare that number with the predicted number using a 95 percent prediction interval based on the baseline data. An approximate 95 percent prediction interval is given by 1.96 times the square root of twice the number of drivers with either exactly one accident or exactly two accidents (Finkelstein and Levin, 1990). If the observed number is found to differ markedly from the predicted number, there are grounds to reject the starting assumption that driving conditions and habits remained the same. See the section Statistical Analyses in Appendix A for further discussion of risk-based allocation.

tion of the data and then use of the model to predict responses for high-risk patients is not equivalent to extrapolation of the data into some unknown region of the sample data. Second, the model can be validated with the observed data, which increases confidence in the model over the unobserved data. Third, the effect of extrapolation is accurately reflected by the standard errors, but the effect is not some wild inflation into unknown territory. This third assumption is an important one, and identification of the appropriate model must be accomplished before a risk-based trial can be undertaken. Once the necessary model is developed, there are no other hidden assumptions. The reliability of the available data is important to this approach.

A clinical example from Finkelstein, Levin, and Robbins (1996b) is given in Box 2-7. That example uses a simple linear model to relate how much the level of total serum cholesterol was reduced from the baseline to the end of follow-up on the basis of a preliminary measurement of the cholesterol level among a group of cholesteremic, sedentary men in the placebo arm of a well-known randomized trial of the cholesterol-lowering compound cholestyramine. If the trial had been designed as a risk-based allocation trial, the actually observed lowering of the cholesterol level among the highest-risk (the most cholesteremic) men given the active drug could have been compared on the basis of a simple linear model with the lowering predicted

BOX 2-7
Potential Effectiveness of Replacing Randomized Allocation with Risk-Based (Assured) Allocation (in Which All Higher Risk Participants Receive the New Treatment)

High levels of cholesterol (at least the low-density lipoprotein component) are generally regarded as a risk factor for heart disease. A primary prevention trial was conducted in which 337 participants were randomly assigned to treatment arms to evaluate the ability of cholestyramine to lower total plasma cholesterol levels. The group with high cholesterol levels (> 290 mg/dl) had an average reduction of 34.42 mg/dl with a treatment effect (the reduction in the cholestyramine-treated high cholesterol subgroup minus the reduction in the high-cholesterol placebo controls) of 29.40 ± 3.77 mg/dl (standard error) (Lipid Research Clinical Program, 1984). The results also suggest that the drug is less effective in absolute terms for participants with lower initial total plasma cholesterol levels (<290 mg/dl). By applying a risk-based allocation model to the same data, the treatment effect is estimated for participants at higher risk (>290 mg of total plasma cholesterol/dl) to be 30.76 ±8.02 mg/dl, which is close to the result of the RCT of 29.40 mg/dl. Thus, for the high-risk patients, the results from the trial with a risk-based allocation design are virtually identical to those of the trial with the conventional design (Finkelstein, Levin, and Robbins, 1996b).

for the same men while they were receiving a placebo. The example illustrates that the risk-based approach would have arrived at the same estimate of treatment effect for those at higher risk as the RCT did.

Some cautions must be observed when risk-based allocation is used. The population of participants entering a trial with a risk-based allocation design should be the same as that for which the model was validated so that the form of the assumed model is correct. Clinicians enrolling patients into the trial need to be comfortable with the allocation rule, because protocol violations raise difficulties just as they do in RCTs. Finally, the standard error of estimates will reflect the effect of extrapolation of the model predictions for the higher-risk patients on the basis of the data for the lower-risk patients. Because of this, a randomized design with balanced arms will have smaller standard errors than a risk-based design with the same number of patients. In the example of the study of cholestyramine in Box 2-7, the standard error was slightly more than doubled for the risk-based design than for the randomized design.

What do these ideas have to do with small clinical trials? Consider the example of bone mineral density loss among astronauts. An obvious risk factor that correlates with bone mineral density loss is the duration of the mission in space: the longer the mission, the greater the bone mineral density loss. What would be required in a risk-based study design is the mathematical form of this relationship for some standard countermeasures (countermeasure is the term that the National Aeronautics and Space Administration uses for a preventive or therapeutic intervention that mitigates bone mineral density loss or other physiological adaptations to long-duration space travel). Astronauts who will be on extended future missions on the International Space Station will be at higher-risk than those who have shorter stays. If those on the longer missions (who are at higher risk) were to receive new experimental countermeasures, their bone mineral density losses could be compared on a case-by-case basis to a prediction of what their bone mineral density loss would have been by use of the standard countermeasures. Such comparisons of observed versus expected or predicted outcomes are familiar in other studies with small sample sizes, such as studies searching for associations of rare cancer with a variety of toxic exposures.

Finally, any trial conducted in an unblinded manner has a potential bias. In some cases a trial with a risk-based allocation design need not be conducted in an unblinded manner; for example, patients may be assured of receiving an active experimental treatment together with a placebo standard treatment if they are at high risk or a placebo experimental treatment together with an active standard treatment if they are lower risk. The trial may be conducted in a blinded manner if the risk measure is not obvious to the patient. In many cases, however, the trial, such as a surgical intervention trial, would have to be unblinded. The issue is nothing new. Solid endpoints unaffected by investigator bias and careful protocols for permitted concomitant behavior are the best safeguard in unblinded trials.

SUMMARY

Scientific research has a long history of well-established, well-documented, and validated methods for the design, conduct, and analysis of clinical trials. A study design that is appropriate includes one with a sufficient sample size and statistical power and proper control of bias to allow a meaningful interpretation of the results. **The committee strongly reaffirms that, whenever feasible, clinical trials should be designed and performed so that they have adequate statistical power.**

When the clinical context does not provide a sufficient number of research participants for a trial with adequate statistical power but the research question has great clinical significance, the committee understands that, by necessity for the advancement of human health, research will proceed. Bearing in mind the statistical power, precision, and validity limitations of studies with small sample sizes, the committee notes that there are innovative design and analysis approaches that can improve the quality of such trials. In small clinical trials, it is more likely that the sample population will share several unique characteristics, for example, disease, exposures, or environment. Thus, it might be more practical in some small clinical trials than in large clinical trials to involve the participants in the design of the trial. By doing so, the investigator can increase the likelihood of compliance, adherence to the regimen, and willingness to participate in monitoring and follow-up activities. Investigators should also keep in mind opportunities for community discussion and conversation during the conduct and planning of all trials. It is also important for investigators to consider confidentiality and privacy in disseminating the results of studies whose sample populations are easily identified. Investigatiors should also keep in mind opportunities for community discussion and consultation during the planning and conduct of all clinical trials.

RECOMMENDATIONS

Because of the constraints of trials with small sample sizes, for example, trials with participants with unique or rare diseases or health conditions, it is particularly important to define the research questions and select outcome measures that are going to make the best possible use of the available participants while minimizing the risks to those individuals.

RECOMMENDATION: Define the research question. Before undertaking a small clinical trial it is particularly important that the research question be well defined and that outcomes and conditions to be evaluated be selected in a manner that will most likely help clinicians make therapeutic decisions.

RECOMMENDATION: Tailor the design. Careful consideration of alternative statistical design and analysis methods should occur at all stages in the multistep process of planning a clinical trial. When designing a small clinical trial, it is particularly important that the statistical design and analysis methods be customized to address the clinical research question and study population.

Clinical researchers have proposed alternative trial designs, some of which have been applied to small clinical trials. For a smaller trial, when the anticipated effect is not great, researchers may encounter a difficult tension between scientific purity or pragmatic necessity. One approach might be to focus on a simple, streamlined hypothesis (not multiple ones) and choose one means of statistical analysis that does not rely on any complicated models and that can be widely validated. An alternative approach is to choose a model-dependent analysis, effectively surrendering any pretense of model validation, knowing that there will not be enough information to validate the model, a risk that could compromise the scientific validity of the trial.

The committee believes that the research base in this area requires further development. Alternative designs have been proposed in a variety of contexts; however, they have not been adequately examined in the context of small studies.

RECOMMENDATION: More research on alternative designs is needed. Appropriate federal agencies should increase support for expanded theoretical and empirical research on the performances of alternative study designs and analysis methods that can be applied to small studies. Areas worthy of more study may include theory development, simulated and actual testing including comparison of existing and newly developed or modified alternative designs and methods of analysis, simulation models, study of limitations of trials with different sample sizes, and modification of a trial during its conduct.

Because of the limitations of small clinical trials it is especially important that the results be reported with accompanying details about the sample size, sample characteristics, and study design. The details necessary to combine evidence from several related studies, for example, measurement methods, main outcomes, and predictors for individual participants, should be published. There are two reasons for this: first, it allows the clinician to appropriately interpret the data within the clinical context, and second, it paves the way for meta-analysis with other small clinical trials or other future analyses of the study, for example, as part of a sequential design or meta-analysis. In the clinical setting, the consequences might be greater if one misinterprets the results. In the research setting, insufficiently described design strategies and methods diminish the study's value for future analyses.

RECOMMENDATION: Clarify methods in reporting of results of clinical trials. In reporting the results of a small clinical trial, with its inherent limitations, it is particularly important to carefully describe all sample characteristics and methods of data collection and analysis for synthesis of the data from the research.

3
Statistical Approaches to Analysis of Small Clinical Trials

A necessary companion to a well-designed clinical trial is its appropriate statistical analysis. Assuming that a clinical trial will produce data that could reveal differences in effects between two or more interventions, statistical analyses are used to determine whether such differences are real or are due to chance. Data analysis for small clinical trials in particular must be focused. In the context of a small clinical trial, it is especially important for researchers to make a clear distinction between preliminary evidence and confirmatory data analysis. When the sample population is small, it is important to gather considerable preliminary evidence on related subjects before the trial is conducted to define the size needed to determine a critical effect. It may be that statistical hypothesis testing is premature. Thus, testing of a null hypothesis might be particularly challenging in the context of a small clinical trial. Thus, in some cases it might be important to focus on evidence rather than to test a hypothesis (Royall, 1997). This is because a small clinical trial is less likely to be self-contained, providing all of the necessary evidence to effectively test a particular hypothesis. Instead, it might be necessary to summarize all of the evidence from the trial and combine it with other evidence available from other trials or laboratory studies. A single large clinical trial is often insufficient to answer a biomedical research question, and it is even more unlikely that a single small clinical trial can do so. Thus, analyses of data must consider the limitations of the

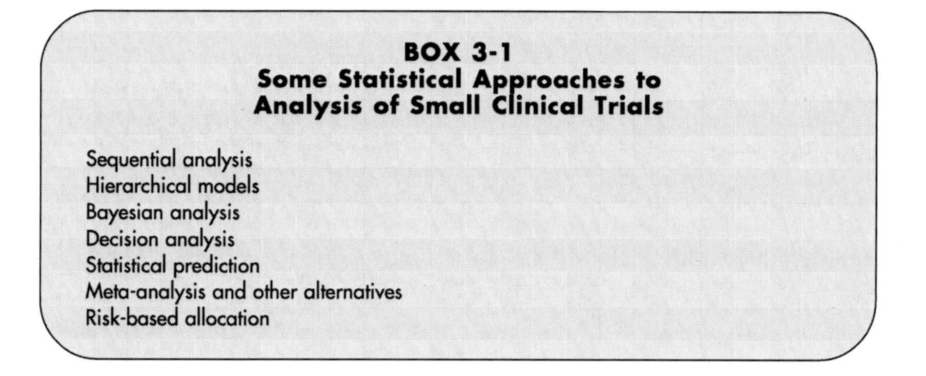
BOX 3-1
Some Statistical Approaches to Analysis of Small Clinical Trials

Sequential analysis
Hierarchical models
Bayesian analysis
Decision analysis
Statistical prediction
Meta-analysis and other alternatives
Risk-based allocation

data at hand and their context in comparison with those of other similar or related studies.

Since data analysis for small clinical trials inevitably involves a number of assumptions, it is logical that several different statistical analyses be conducted. If these analyses give consistent results under different assumptions, one can be more confident that the results are not due to unwarranted assumptions. In general, certain types of analyses (see Box 3-1) are more amenable to small studies. Each is briefly described in the sections that follow.

SEQUENTIAL ANALYSIS

Sequential analysis refers to an analysis of the data as they accumulate, with a view toward stopping the study as soon as the results become statistically compelling. This is in contrast to a sequential design (see Chapter 2), in which the probability that a participant is assigned to a particular intervention is changed depending on the accumulating results. In sequential analysis the probabilty of assignment to an intervention is constant across the study.

Sequential analysis methods were first used in the context of industrial quality control in the late 1920s (Dodge and Romig, 1929). The use of sequential analysis in clinical trials has been extensively described by Armitage (1975), Heitjan (1997), and Whitehead (1999). Briefly, the data are analyzed as the results for each participant are obtained. After each observation, the decision is made to (1) continue the study by enrolling additional participants, (2) stop the study with the conclusion that there is a statistically significant difference between the treatments, or (3) stop the study and conclude that there is not a statistically significant difference between the interventions. The boundaries for the decision-making process are constructed by using considerations of power and size needed to determine an effect size similar to those used to determine sample size (see, for example Whitehead [1999]). Commercially available software can be used to construct the boundaries.

In sequential analysis, the final sample size is not known at the beginning of the study. On average, sequential analysis will lead to a smaller average sample size than that in an equivalently powered study with a fixed-sample-size design. This is a major advantage to sequential analysis and is a reason that it should be given consideration when one is planning and analyzing a small clinical trial. For example, take the case study of sickle cell disease introduced in Chapter 1 and consider the analysis of the clinical design problem introduced in Box 1-4 as an example of sequential analysis (Box 3-2).

Data from a clinical trial accumulate gradually over a period of time that can extend to months or even years. Thus, results for patients recruited early in the study are available for interpretation while patients are still being recruited and allocated to treatment. This feature allows the emerging evidence to be used to decide when to stop the study. In particular, it may be desirable to stop the study if a clear treatment difference is apparent, thereby avoiding the allocation of further patients to the less successful therapy. Investigators may also want to stop a study that no longer has much chance of demonstrating a treatment difference (Whitehead, 1992, 1997).

For example, consider the analysis of an intervention (countermeasure) to prevent the loss of bone mineral density in sequentially treated groups of astronauts resulting from their exposure to microgravity during space travel (Figure 3-1). The performance index is the bone mineral density (in grams per square centimeter) of the calcaneus. S refers to success, where p is the probability of success and p^* is the cumulative mean. F refers to failure, where q is the probability of failure and q^* is the cumulative mean. The confidence intervals for p and q are obtained after each space mission, that is, for p, (p_1, p_2), and for q, (q_1, q_2). The sequential accumulation of data then allows one to accept the countermeasure if p_1 is greater than p^* and q_2 is less than q^* or reject the countermeasure if p_2 is less than p^* or q_1 is greater than q^*. Performance indices will be acceptable when success S, a gain or mild loss, occurs on at least 75 percent ($p^* = 0.75$) of the cases (astronaut missions) and when F, severe bone mineral density loss, occurs in no more than 5 percent ($q^* = 0.05$) of the cases. Unacceptable performance indices occur with less than a 75 percent success rate or more than a 5 percent failure rate. As the number of performance indices increases, level 1 performance crite-

BOX 3-2
Clinical Trial for Treatment of Sickle Cell Disease

Sickle Cell disease is a red blood cell (RBC) disorder that affects 1 in 200 African Americans. Fifty percent of individuals living with sickle cell disease die before age 40. The most common complications include stroke, renal failure, and chronic severe pain. Patients who have a stroke are predisposed to having another one.

Mixed donor and host stem cell chimerism (e.g., the recipient patient has stem cells of her or his own origin and also those from the transplant donor) is curative for sickle cell disease. Only 20 percent of donor RBC production (and 80 percent of recipient RBC production) is required to cure the abnormality. Conditioning of the recipient is required for the transplanted bone marrow stem cells to become established. The degree of HLA (human leukocyte antigen) mismatch as well as the sensitization state (i.e., chronic transfusion immunizes the recipient) influences how much conditioning is required to establish 20 percent donor chimerism.

In patients who have an HLA-identical donor and who have not been heavily transfused, 200 centigrays (cGy) of total body irradiation (TBI) is sufficient to establish donor engraftment (establish a cure). This dose of irradiation has been shown to be well tolerated. In heavily transfused recipients who are HLA mismatched, more conditioning will probably be required. The optimal dose of TBI for this cohort has not been established. The focus of this study is to establish the optimum dose of TBI to achieve 20 percent donor cells (chimerism) in patients enrolled in the protocol.

How many patients must be enrolled per cohort to obtain durable bone marrow stem cell establishment (engraftment)? Patients are monitored monthly for the level of donor chimerism. Engraftment can be considered durable if 20 percent donor chimerism is present at ≥6 months. When can TBI dose escalation be implemented? How many patients are required per group before an increase in dose can be made?

Cohort	Number of subjects needed	TBI dose (cGy)
A	to be determined (see below)	200
B	"	250
C	"	300
D	"	350

One traditional approach to this problem is to identify an acceptable engraftment rate and to then identify the number of subjects required to ensure that the confidence interval for the true proportion is sufficiently narrow to be protective of human health. For example, if the desired engraftment rate is 95 percent, 19 subjects will provide a 95 percent confidence interval with a width of 10 percent (i.e., 0.85 to 1.00). If for a particular application, this interval is too wide, a width of 5 percent can be obtained with 73 subjects (0.90 to 1.00).

On the basis of these results, should 73 subjects be required for each TBI dose group? Is a total of 292 patients really needed for all dose groups? The answer is that a much smaller total number of patients is required by invoking a simple sequential testing strategy. For example, assume that the study begins with three patients in the lowest-dose group and it is observed that none of the patients are cured. On the basis of a binomial distribution and by use of a target engraftment proportion of 0.95, the probability that zero of three engraftments will be established when the true population

continues

proportion is 0.95 is approximately 1 in 10,000. Similarly, the cumulative probability of one or fewer cures is less than 15 percent. As such, after only three patients are tested, considerable information regarding whether the true cure rate is 95 percent or more is already available. Following this simple sequential strategy, one would test each dose (beginning with the lowest dose) with a small number of patients (e.g., three patients) and increase to the next dose level if the results of the screening trial indicate that the probability of cure for the targeted proportion (e.g., 0.95 percent) is small. In the current example, one would clearly increase the dose if zero of three patients was cured and would most likely increase the dose to the next level even if one or two patients were cured. If, in this example, all three patients engrafted, one would then test either 19 or 73 patients (depending on the desired width of the confidence interval) and determine a confidence interval for the true engraftment rate with the desired level of precision. If the upper confidence limit is less than the targeted engraftment rate, then one would proceed to the next highest TBI dose level and repeat the test.

ria can be set; for example, *S* is equal to a gain or no worse than 1 percent loss of bone mineral density relative to that at baseline. Indeterminate (*I*) is equal to a moderate loss of 1 to 2 percent from that at the baseline. *F* is equal to the severe loss of 2 percent or more from that at the baseline (Feiveson, 2000). See Box 1-2 for an alternate design discussion of this case study.

The use of study stopping (cessation) rules that are based on successive examinations of accumulating data may cause difficulties because of the need to reconcile such stopping rules with the standard approach to statistical analysis used for the analysis of data from most clinical trials. This standard approach is known as the "frequentist approach." In this approach the analysis takes a form that is dependent on the study design. When such analyses assume a design in which all data are simultaneously available, it is called a "fixed-sample analysis." If the data from a clinical trial are not examined until the end of the study, then a fixed-sample analysis is valid. In comparison, if the data are examined in a way that might lead to early cessation of the study or to some other change of design, then a fixed-sample analysis will not be valid. The lack of validity is a matter of degree: if early cessation or a change of design is an extremely remote possibility, then fixed-sample methods will be approximately valid (Whitehead, 1992, 1997).

For example, in a randomized clinical trial for investigation of the effect of a selenium nutritional supplement on the prevention of skin cancer, it is determined that plasma selenium levels are not rising as expected in some patients in the supplemented group, indicating a possible noncompliance problem. In this case, the failure of some subjects to receive the prescribed amount of selenium supplement would have led to a loss of power to detect a significant benefit, if one was present. One could then initiate a prestudy

A

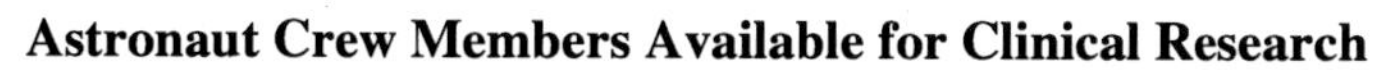

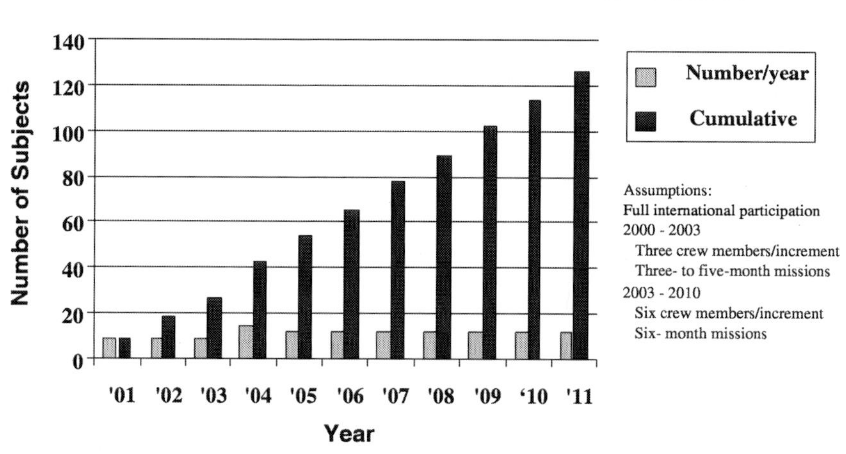

B

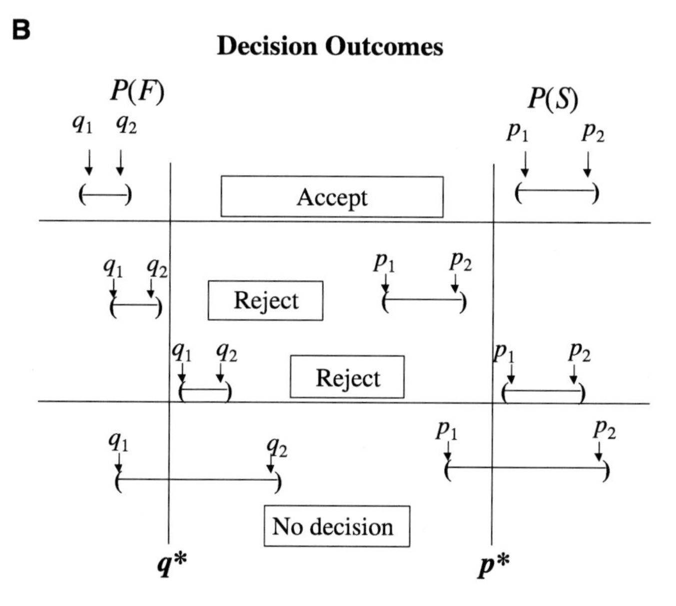

FIGURE 3-1 Parameters for a clinical trial with a sequential design for prevention of loss of bone mineral density in astronauts. A. Group sample sizes available for clinical study. B. Establishment of repeated confidence intervals for a clinical intervention for prevention of loss of bone mineral density for determination of the success (*S*) or failure (*F*) of the intervention.

SOURCE: Feiveson (2000).

BOX 3-3
Sequential Testing with Limited Resources

As an illustration of sequential testing in small clinical studies, consider the innovative approach to forensic drug testing proposed by Hedayat, Izenman, and Zhang (1996). Suppose that *N* units such as pills or tablets or squares of lysergic acid diethylamide (LSD) are obtained during an arrest and one would like to determine the minimal number that would have to be screened to state with 95 percent confidence that at least N_1 of the total *N* samples will be positive. To solve the problem, define *m* as the expected number of negative units in the initial random sample of *n* units and *X* as the observed number of negative units in a sample of size *n*. Typically, the forensic scientist assumes that *m* is equal to 0, *n* samples are collected, and the actual number of negative samples (*X*) is determined. Next, define *k* as the minimum number of positive drug samples that are needed to achieve a conviction in the case. One wishes to test with a confidence of 100(1 − α, where α is the probability of committing a type 1 error) percent that $N_1 \geq k$. The question is: what is the smallest sample size *n* needed?

Hedayat and co-workers showed that the problem can be described in terms of the inequality

$max_{N1<k} \text{Prob}[X \leq m \mid N_1] \leq \alpha,$

which is equivalent to

$max_{N1 \leq k-1} \text{Prob}[X \leq m \mid N_1] \leq \alpha,$

and is satisfied by

$\text{Prob}[X \leq m \mid N_1 = k - 1] \leq \alpha.$

This is a cumulative probability of the hypergeometric distribution, that can be expressed as

$$\sum_{i=n-m}^{n} = \frac{\binom{k-1}{i}\binom{N-k+1}{n-i}}{\binom{N}{n}} \alpha.$$

treatment period in which potential noncompliers could be identified and eliminated from the study before randomization (Jennison and Turnbull, 1983).

Another reason for early examination of study results is to check the assumptions made when designing the trial. For example, in an experiment where the primary response variable is quantitative, the sample size is often set assuming this variable to be normally distributed with a certain variance. For binary response data, sample size calculations rely on an assumed value for the background incidence rate; for time-to-event data when individuals enter the trial at staggered intervals, an estimate of the subject accrual rate is important in determining the appropriate accrual period. An early interim

For example, assume that the total number of units under investigation is 150 and suppose that one wants to claim with 95 percent confidence that the number of positive units, N_1, is at least 135. If one assumes that there will be no negative units in the initial sample (i.e., $m = 0$) then one can begin with an initial sample of 25, using the inequality given above. The investigators draw a random sample of 25, and if no negative units are found, the investigators can conclude with 95 percent confidence that the total number of positive units (N_1) is greater than 135. Note that if one actually observes X to be equal to 1 negative unit, one then can determine what value of N_1 is feasible or recompute n. For example, say that one observes X is equal to 2 negative units among 25 initial samples. With 95 percent confidence one can claim that k equal to 118 positive units will be found. Alternatively, if one requires N_1 to be ≥ 135 positive units, one can increase n to 61 samples by drawing an additional 61 - 25 = 36 random samples.

A useful example in clinical trials is the comparison of a new drug with a standard drug for the treatment of a rare disease. For example, it may be known that the rate of response to an existing drug is 80 percent; however, the drug has serious side effects. A new drug without the side effect profile of the old drug has been developed, but it is not known whether it is equally efficacious. Power computations revealed that 150 subjects are required to document that the response rate is at least 90 percent with 95 percent confidence (i.e., at least 135 of 150 patients respond). Unfortunately, 150 subjects are not available. Using the strategy developed by Hedayat and colleagues (1996), one can examine 25 patients, and if they all respond, then one can conclude with 95 percent confidence that the total number of responders is at least 135 among the 150 patients that the investigators would have liked to test. There are numerous applications of this type of sequential testing strategy in small clinical trials.

analysis can reveal inaccurate assumptions in time for adjustments to be made to the design (Jennison and Turnbull, 1983).

Sequential methods typically lead to savings in sample size, time, and cost compared with those for standard fixed-sample procedures (Box 3-3). However, continuous monitoring is not always practical.

HIERARCHICAL MODELS

Hierarchical models can be quite useful in the context of small clinical trials in two regards. First, hierarchical models provide a natural framework for combining information from a series of small clinical trials conducted within ecological units (e.g., space missions or clinics). In the case where the data are complete, in which the same response measure is available for each individual, hierarchical models provide a more rigorous solution than meta-analysis, in that there is no reason to use effect magnitudes as the unit of observation. Note, however, that a price must be paid (i.e., the total sample size must be increased) to reconstruct a larger trial out of a series of smaller trials. Second, hierarchical models also provide a foundation for analysis of longitudinal studies, which are necessary for increasing the power of research involving small clinical trials. By repeatedly obtaining data for the same subject over time as part of a study of a single treatment or a crossover study, the total number of subjects required in the trial is reduced. The reduction in the sample size number is proportional to the degree of independence of the repeated measurements.

A common theme in medical research is two-stage sampling, that is, sampling of responses within experimental units (e.g., patients) and sampling of experimental units within populations. For example, in prospective longitudinal studies patients are repeatedly sampled and assessed in terms of a variety of endpoints such as mental and physical levels of functioning or in terms of the response of one or more biological systems to one or more forms of treatment. These patients are in turn sampled from a population, often stratified on the basis of treatment delivery, for example, in a clinic, in a hospital, or during space missions. Like all biological and behavioral characteristics, the outcome measures exhibit individual differences. Investigators should be interested in not only the mean response pattern but also the distribution of these response patterns (e.g., time trends) in the population of patients. One can then address the number or proportion of patients who are functioning more or less positively at a specific rate. One can then describe the treatment-outcome relationship not as a fixed law but as a family of laws, the parameters of which describe the individual biobehavioral tendencies of the subjects in the population (Bock, 1983). This view of biological and behavioral research may lead to Bayesian methods of data analysis. The relevant distributions exist objectively and can be investigated empirically.

In medical research, a typical example of two-stage sampling is the longitudinal clinical trial, in which patients are randomly assigned to different treatments and are repeatedly evaluated over the course of the study. Despite recent advances in statistical methods for longitudinal research, the cost of medical research is not always commensurate with the quality of the analyses. Reports of such studies often consist of little more than an endpoint analysis in which measurements only for those participants who have completed the study are considered in the analysis or the last available measurement for each participant is carried forward as if all participants had, in fact, completed the study. In the first example of a "completer- only" analysis, the available sample at the end of the study may have little similarity to the sample initially randomized. There is some improvement in the case of carrying the last observation forward. However, participants treated in the analysis as if they have had identical exposures to the drug may have quite different exposures in reality or their experiences while receiving the drug may be complicated by other factors that led to their withdrawal from the study but that are ignored in the analysis. Both cases lead to dramatic losses of statistical power since the measurements made on the intermediate occasions are simply discarded. In these studies a review of the typical level of intraindividual variability of responses should raise serious questions regarding reliance on any single measurement.

To illustrate the problem, consider the following example. Suppose a longitudinal randomized clinical trial is conducted to study the effects of a particular therapeutic intervention (countermeasure) on bone mineral density measurements taken at multiple points in time during the course of a space mission. At the end of the study, the data comprise a file of bone mineral density measurements for each patient (astronaut) in each treatment group. In addition to the usual completer or end-point analysis, a data analyst might compute means for each week and might fit separately for each group a linear or curvilinear trend line that shows average bone mineral density loss per week. A more sophisticated analyst might fit the line using some variant of the Potthoff-Roy procedure, although this would require complete and similarly time-structured data for all subjects (Bock, 1979).

Despite the question of whether bone mineral density measurements are related to the ability of an astronaut to function in space, most objectionable is the representation of the mean trend in the population as a biological relationship acting within individual subjects. The analysis might purport that as any astronaut uses a countermeasure he or she will decrease the effect of life in a weightless environment on bone mineral density loss at some fixed rate (e.g., 0.1 percent per week). This is a gross oversimplification. The account is somewhat improved by reporting of mean trends for important subgroups: astronauts of various ages, males and females, and so on. Even then, within such groups some patients will respond more to a given countermeasure, some will respond less, and the responses of others will not change at all. Like all biological characteristics, there are individual differences in response trends. Therefore, both the mean trend and the distribution of trends in the population of patients are of interest. One can then speak of the number or proportion of patients who respond to a clinically acceptable degree and the rates at which their biological status changes over time.

In a longitudinal study, repeated observations are nested within individuals and the hierarchical model is used to incorporate the effects of intrasubject correlation on estimates of uncertainty (i.e., standard errors and confidence intervals) and tests of hypotheses for the fixed effects or structural parameters (e.g., differential treatment efficacy) in the model. Note that hierarchical models are equally useful in the context of clustered data, in which participants are nested within groups (e.g., different studies or space missions), and the sharing of this similar environment induces a correlation among the responses of participants within strata.

Analysis of this type of data (under the assumptions that a subset of the regression parameters has a distribution in the population of participants and that the model residuals have a distribution in the population of responses within participants and also in the population of participants) belongs to the class of statistical analytical models called:

- mixed model (Elston and Grizzle, 1962; Longford, 1987);
- regression with randomly dispersed parameters (Rosenberg, 1973);
- exchangeability between multiple regressions (Lindley and Smith, 1972);
- two-stage stochastic regression, (Fearn, 1975);
- James-Stein estimation (James and Stein, 1961);
- variance component models (Dempster, Rubin, and Tsutakawa, 1981; Harville, 1977);
- random coefficient models (DeLeeuw and Kreft, 1986);
- hierarchical linear models (Bryk and Raudenbush, 1987);
- multilevel models (Goldstein, 1986); and
- random-effect regression models (Laird and Ware, 1982).

Along with the seminal articles that have described these statistical models, several book-length texts that further describe these methods have been published (Bock, 1989; Bryk and Raudenbush, 1992; Diggle, Liang, and Zeger, 1994; Goldstein, 1995; Jones, 1993; Lindsey, 1993; Longford, 1993). For the most part, these treatments are based on the assumptions that the residual effects are normally distributed with zero means and a covariance

BOX 3-4
Power Consideration for Space Mission Clinical Trials

A natural application for hierarchical regression models is the problem in which astronauts are nested within space missions and the intervention (e.g., the presence or the absence of a particular countermeasure) is randomly assigned at the level of the space mission. To illustrate the problem, assume that one is interested in detecting a difference of a 0.5 standard deviation unit between control and experimental conditions by a one-tailed test. In addition, assume that five astronauts are available per space mission and that the intraspace mission correlation is 0.2.

Assuming a Type I error rate of 5 percent (i.e., 95 percent confidence), how many space missions are required to have 80 percent statistical power of detection of a difference? Using statistical power computations for the clustered *t* distribution (Hsieh, 1988) one finds that detection of a difference of 0.5 standard deviation unit with 80 percent power would require for each condition (i.e., the control versus the experimental condition) 18 space missions, each with 5 subjects, or a total of 180 astronauts.Note that if the effect size is increased to a difference of 1 standard deviation unit, which may be acceptable for bone mineral density measurement data, the number of space missions is reduced to 5 per condition, for a total of 50 astronauts. In a longitudinal study (i.e., repeated evaluation of astronauts during their tour of duty), statistical power computations become more complex because they can involve both random effects and residual autocorrelations. (The interested reader is referred to the paper by Hedeker, Gibbons, and Waternaux [1999]).

matrix in all participants, and that the random effects are normally distributed with zero means and covariance matrix. Recent review articles summarize the use of hierarchical models in biostatistics and health services research (Gibbons, 2000; Gibbons and Hedeker, 2000). Some statistical details of the general linear hierarchical regression model are provided in Appendix A. The case study presented in Box 3-4 provides an example of how hierarchical models can be used to aid in the design and analysis of small clinical trials.

BAYESIAN ANALYSIS

The majority of statistical techniques that clinical investigators encounter are of the frequentist school and are characterized by significance levels, confidence intervals, and concern over the bias of estimates (Jennison and Turnbull, 1983). The Bayesian philosophy of statistical inference however is fundamentally different from that underlying the frequentist approach (Malakoff, 1999; Thall, 2000). In certain types of investigations Bayesian analysis can lead to practical methods that are similar to those used by statisticians who use the frequentist approach.

The Bayesian approach has a subjective element. It focuses on an unknown parameter value q, which measures the effect of the experimental treatment. Before designing a study or collecting any data, the investigator acquires all available information about the activities of both the experimental and the control treatments. This provides some information about the possible value of θ.

> The Bayesian approach is based on the supposition that the investigator's opinion can be expressed in the form of a value for $P(\theta \leq x)$ for every x between $-\infty$ and ∞. Here $P(\theta \leq x)$ represents the probability that θ is less than or equal to x. The probability is not frequentist: it does not represent the proportion of times that θ is less than or equal to x. Instead, $P(\theta \leq x)$ represents how likely the investigator *thinks* it to be that θ is less than or equal to x. The investigator is allowed to think only in terms of functions $P(\theta \leq x)$ which rise from 0 at $x = -\infty$ to 1 at $x = \infty$. Thus $P(\theta \leq x)$ defines a probability distribution for θ_1, which will be called the *subjective distribution* of θ. Notice how deep the division between the frequentist and the Bayesian goes: even the notion of probability receives a different interpretation (Jennison and Turnbull, 1983, p. 203).

Thus, before the investigator has observed any data, a subjective distribution of θ can be formulated from the experiences and knowledge gained by others. At this stage, the subjective distribution can be called the *prior distribution* of θ. After data are collected, these will influence and change opinions about θ. The assessment of where q lies may change (reflected by a change in the location of the subjective distribution), and uncertainty about its value should decrease (reflected by a decrease in the spread of this subjective distribution). The combination of observed data and prior opinion is governed by Bayes's theorem, which provides an automatic update of the investigator's subjective opinion. The theorem then specifies a new subjective distribution for θ, called a *posterior distribution* (Jennison and Turnbull, 1983).

The attraction of the Bayesian approach lies in its simplicity of concept and the directness of its conclusions. Its flexibility and lack of concern for interim inspections are especially valuable in sequential clinical trials. The main problem with the Bayesian approach, however, lies in the idea of a subjective distribution.

> Subjective opinions are a legitimate part of personal inferences. A small investigating team might be in sufficient agreement to share the same prior distribution but it is less likely that all members of the team will hold the same prior opinions and some members will be reluctant to accept an analysis based in part on opinions that they do not share. An alternative possibility is for investi-

gators to adopt a prior distribution representing only vague subjective opinion, which is quickly overwhelmed by information from the data. The latter suggestion leads to analyses which are similar to frequentist inferences, but it would appear to lose the spirit of the Bayesian approach. If the prior distribution is not a true representation of subjective opinion then neither is the posterior (Jennison and Turnbull, 1983, p. 204).

More generally, the Bayesian approach has the following advantages:

- **Problem formulation.** Many problems, such as inferences or decision making based on small amounts of data, are easy to formulate and solve by Bayesian methods.
- **Sequential analysis.** Because the posterior distribution can be updated repeatedly, using each successive posterior distribution as the prior distribution for the next update, it is the natural paradigm for sequential decision making.
- **Meta-analysis.** Bayesian hierarchical models provide a natural framework for combining information from different sources. This is often referred to as "meta-analysis" in the context of clinical trials, but the methods are quite broadly applicable.
- **Prediction.** An especially useful tool is the predictive probability of a future event. This allows one to make statements such as "Given that an astronaut has not suffered bone mineral density loss during the first year of a 2-year space mission, the probability that he or she will suffer bone mineral density loss during the second year is 25 percent."
- **Communication.** Bayesian models, methods, and inferences are often easier to communicate to nonstatisticians. This is because most people think and behave like Bayesians, whether or not they understand or are even aware of the formal paradigm. The posterior distribution provides a framework for describing and communicating one's conclusions in a variety of ways that make sense to nonstatisticians. Although the details are not presented here, Bayesian methods (Thall, 2000; Thall and Sung, 1998; Thall and Russell, 1998; Thall, Simon, and Estey, 1995; Thall, Simon, and Shen, 2000; Whitehead and Brunier, 1995) can be applied in most of the design and analysis situations described in this report and in many cases will be extremely useful for the analysis of results of small clinical trials.

DECISION ANALYSIS

Decision analysis is a modeling technique that systematically considers all possible management options for a problem (Hillner and Centor, 1987). It uses probabilities and utilities to explicitly define decisions. The computational methods allow one to evaluate the importance of any variable in the decision-masking process. Sensitivity analysis describes the process of recalculating the analysis as one changes a variable through a series of plausible values. The steps to be taken in decision analysis are outlined in Table 3-1.

As mentioned in Chapter 2, one can use decision analysis as an aid in the experimental design process. If one models a clinical situation a priori, one can test the importance of a single value in making the decision in question. Performance of a sensitivity analysis before a study is designed to provide an understanding of the influence of a given value on the decision. Such analyses can determine the best use of a small clinical trial. This pre-analysis allows one to focus data collection on important variables (see Box 3-5).

The other major advantage of decision analysis occurs after data collection. If one assumes that the sample size is inadequate and therefore that the confidence intervals on the effect in question are wide, one may still have a clinical situation for which a decision is required. One might have to make decisions under conditions of uncertainty, despite a desire to increase the certainty. The use of decision analysis can make explicit the uncertain decision, even informing the level of confidence in the decision. A 1990 Institute of Medicine report states: it is this flexibility of decision analysis that gives it the potential to help set priorities for clinical investigation and effective transfer of research findings to clinical practice (Institute of Medicine, 1990). The formulation of a decision analytical model helps investigators consider which health outcomes are important and how important they are to one another. Decision analysis also facilitates consideration of the potential marginal benefit of a new intervention by forcing comparisons with other alternatives or "fallback positions." Combining several methodologies, such as

TABLE 3-1 Steps in a Decision Analysis

- Frame the question
- Establish a time horizon
- Structure the decision tree (choices, chances, outcomes)
- Assess the probabilities
- Assess the utilities
- Evaluate the decision tree (expected value)
- Perform sensitivity analysis
- Interpret the results
- Iterate

SOURCE: Pauker (2000).

BOX 3-5
Using Decision Analysis to Prevent Osteoporosis in Space

Consider a decision analysis that takes the following into consideration:

- a long space mission accelerates bone mineral density loss,
- bone mineral density loss can produce fractures now or in the future,
- fractures produce disabilities now and disabilities in the future, and
- a proposed special program may have efficacy in ameliorating bone mineral density loss, but may have side effects.

Determine the expectation by evaluating a decision tree (Figure 3.2). A decision tree can be set up for either a surrogate measure of bone loss (e.g., bone mineral density loss) or for an actual disabling outcome (e.g., bone fracture, as illustrated in Figure 3.3).

Then by making a number of assumptions, such as

- probability of fracture (*p*) = 0.2,
- efficacy of special program (*e*) = 0.3,
- probability of side effects (*s*) = 0.05,
- quality of life (*LT*) after fracture (*qFx*) = 0.85,
- quality of life (*LT*) after side effects (*qSE*) = 0.999,
- life expectancy of astronaut (*LE*) = 35 *y*, where *y* is years,
- short-term morbidity fracture (*stmFx*) = 0.3 *y*,
- short-term morbidity side effects (*stmSE*) = 0.1 *y*, and
- short-term morbidity special program (*stmSP*) = 0.04 *y*

one can assign values at the chance nodes to pick the best option (see Figure 3.4).

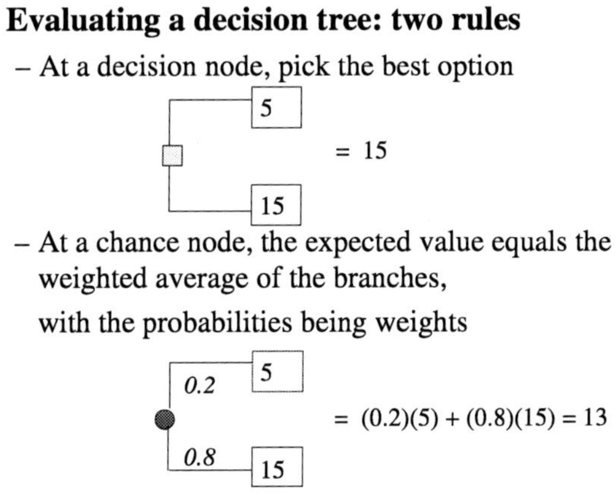

Evaluating a decision tree: two rules

– At a decision node, pick the best option

– At a chance node, the expected value equals the weighted average of the branches,
with the probabilities being weights

FIGURE 3-2 Decision analysis expectation. SOURCE: Pauker (2000).

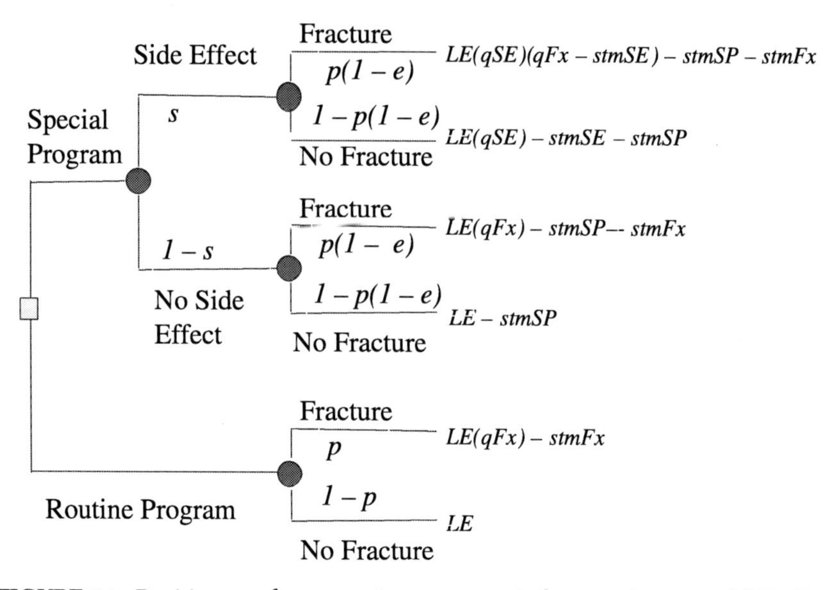

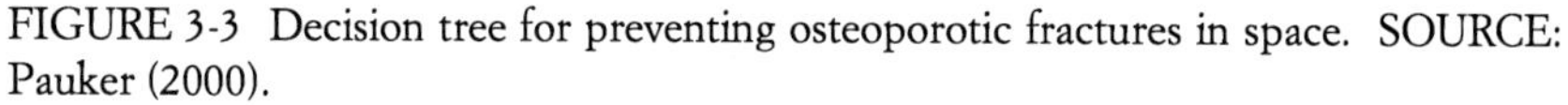
FIGURE 3-3 Decision tree for preventing osteoporotic fractures in space. SOURCE: Pauker (2000).

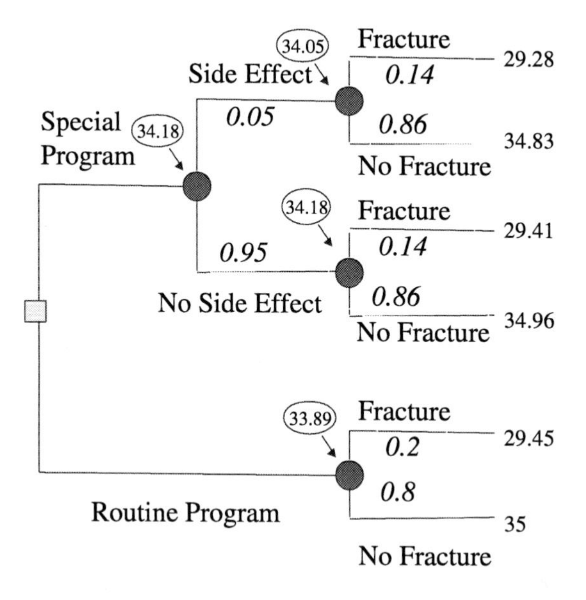

FIGURE 3-4 Assigning values at chance nodes to pick the best option (clinical intervention) for preventing osteoporotic fractures in space. SOURCE: Pauker (2000).

decision analysis, with a sequential clinical trials approach potentially offers additional improvements in the means of determining the efficacy of a therapeutic intervention in small trial populations.

Although decision analysis does not address the questions raised by small clinical trials, it can allow a better trial design to be used and interpretation of the results of such trials.

- Decision analytical models can combine data from diverse sources and examine interactions.
- Decision analytical models are most powerfully used to answer the question "What if?" by sensitivity analyses.
- Decision analytical models can examine the impact of morbidity and effects on quality of life because they can integrate many attributes in a utility structure.
- Decision analyses might be used sequentially in small ongoing trials, in which the results for every additional patient might guide the use of the model for subsequent patients.
- Probability functions such a beta functions can provide such automatic updating of distributions in a model as more patients' experiences are revealed (Pauker, 2000).

STATISTICAL PREDICTION

When the number of control samples is potentially large and the number of experimental samples is small and is obtained sequentially from a series of clusters with small sample sizes (e.g., space missions), traditional comparisons of the aggregate means or medians may be of limited value. In those cases, one can view the problem not as a classical hypothesis testing problem but as a problem of statistical prediction. Conceptualized in that way, the problem is one of deriving a limit or interval on the basis of the control distribution that will include the mean or median for all or a subset of the experimental cluster samples. For example, one may wish to compare the median bone mineral density loss in 5 astronauts in each of five future space missions (i.e., a total of 25 astronauts clustered in groups of 5 each) with the distribution of bone mineral density loss in controls over a similar period of time on Earth or alternatively with that for a control group of astronauts who are in a weightless environment (e.g., the International Space Station) but who are not taking part in a particular countermeasure program. As the number of cluster samples increases, confidence in the decision rule also increases. In the following, a general nonparametric approach to this problem is developed, and its use is illustrated with the problem of testing for bone mineral density loss during space missions. Although more general than parametric alternatives, a loss of statistical power is associated with the nonparametric approach. Parametric alternatives (normal, lognormal, and Poisson distributions) are presented in Appendix A and can be used when the observed data are consistent with one of these distributions.

The prediction problem involves construction of a limit or interval that will contain one or more new measurements drawn from that same distribution with a given level of confidence. As an example, in environmental monitoring problems one may be interested in determining whether a single new measurement (or the mean of n new measurements) obtained from an on-site monitoring location is consistent with background levels as characterized by a series of n measurements obtained from off-site (i.e., background) monitoring locations.

If the new measurement(s) lies within the interval (or below [above] the upper [lower] limit), then one can conclude that the measurement from the on-site monitoring location is consistent with the background measurement and is therefore not affected by activities at the site from which the measurement was obtained. By contrast, if the new measurement(s) lies outside of the interval, one can conclude that it is inconsistent with the background measurement and may potentially have been affected by the activities at the site (e.g., disposal of waste or some industrial process).

One can imagine that as the number of future measurements (i.e., new monitoring locations and number of constituents to be examined) gets large, the prediction interval must expand so that the joint probability of any one of those comparisons by chance alone is small, say 5 percent. Of course, this results in a loss of statistical power. To this end, Gibbons (1987b) and Davis and McNichols (1987) (see Gibbons [1994] for a review) suggested that the new measurements be tested sequentially so that a smaller and more environmentally protective limit can be used. The basic idea is that in the presence of an initial value that exceeds the background level in an on-site monitoring location (initial exceedance), another sample for independent verification of the level should be obtained. A true exceedance is indicated only if both the initial level and the verification resample exceed the limit (or are outside the interval). There are many variations of this sequential strategy in which more than one additional sample (resample) may be obtained. The net result is that a much smaller prediction limit can be used sequentially compared with the limit that would be used if the statistical prediction decision was based on the result of a single comparison, leading to a dramatic increase in statistical power. In fact, this strategy is now used almost exclusively in environmental monitoring programs in the United States (Davis, 1993; Gibbons, 1994, 1996; Environmental Protection Agency, 1992).

This idea can be directly adapted to the problem of loss of bone mineral density in astronauts, particularly with respect to the design and analysis of data from a series of small clinical trials (e.g., space missions, each consisting of a small number of astronauts) and in which a potentially large number of outcomes are simultaneously assessed. To provide a foundation, consider the case in which a study has n control subjects (e.g., astronauts on the International Space Station or in a simulated environment, but without countermeasures) and a series of p replicate experimental cohorts (e.g., space missions), each of size n_i (e.g., $n_i = 5$ astronauts in each of $p = 5$ space missions). The objective is to use the n control measurements to derive an upper (lower) bound for a subset (e.g., 50 percent) of the n_i experimental subjects in at least one of the p experimental subject cohorts (e.g., space missions).

Given the previous characterization of the problem and the questionable distributional form of the outcomes of multiple countermeasures, a natural approach to the solution of this problem is to proceed nonparametrically. For a particular outcome (e.g., bone mineral density), define an upper prediction limit as the uth largest control measurement among the n control subjects. If u is equal to n, the prediction limit is the largest control measurement for that particular outcome measure or endpoint. If u is equal to $n - 1$ then the prediction limit is the second largest control measurement for that outcome measure. A natural advantage of using $u < n$ is that it provides an automatic adjustment for outliers, in that the largest $n - u$ values are removed. Note, however, that the larger the difference between u and n the lower the overall confidence, if everything else is kept equal.

Now consider the experimental subjects. Assume that n_i experimental subjects (e.g., astronauts who are subjected to experimental countermeasures) exist in each of p experimental subject cohorts (e.g., space missions). Let s_i be the number of subjects required to be contained within the interval for cohort i. For example, if n_i is equal to 5 and one wishes to have the median value for cohort i be below the upper prediction limit, then s_i is equal to 3. An effect of the experimental intervention on a particular outcome measure is declared only if the s_ith largest measurement (e.g., the median) lies outside of the prediction interval (or above [below] the prediction limit in the one-sided case) in all p experimental subject cohorts.

The questions of interest are as follows:

1. What is the probability of a chance exceedance in all p experimental subject cohorts for different values of n, u, n_i, s_i, and p?
2. How is this probability affected by various numbers of outcome measures (i.e., k)?
3. What is the power to detect a real difference between control and experimental conditions for a given statistical strategy?

A drawback to this method is that the control group is typically not a concurrent control group. Thus, if other conditions, in addition to the intervention being evaluated, are changed, it will not be possible to determine if the changes are in fact due to the experimental condition.

Specific details regarding implementation of the approach and a general methodology for answering these questions is presented in Appendix A and is illustrated in Box 3-6.

The use of statistical prediction limits described here represents a paradigm shift in the way in which small clinical studies are designed and analyzed. The method involves characterization of the distribution of control measurements and the use of parameters for the control distribution to draw inferences from a series of more limited samples of experimental measurements. This is a classical problem in statistical prediction and departs from the more commonly used paradigm of hypothesis testing. The methodology described here is applicable to virtually any problem in which the number of potential endpoints is large and the number of available subjects is small. In a recent work by Gibbons and colleagues (submitted for publication), a similar approach was developed to compare relatively small numbers of experimental tissues to a larger number of control tissues in terms of potentially thousands of gene expression levels obtained from nucleic acid microarrays. To provide ease of application, they developed a "probability calculator" that computes confidence levels and statistical power for any set of values of n, n_i, p, u, i, s_i, and k. (The probability calculator is freely available at www.uic.edu/labs/biostat/ and is useful for both design and analysis of small clinical studies.)

META-ANALYSIS: SYNTHESIS OF RESULTS OF INDEPENDENT STUDIES

Meta-analysis refers to a set of statistical procedures used to summarize empirical research in the literature (Table 3-2). Although the concept of combining the results of many studies has its origins in the early 1900s agricultural experiments, Glass in 1976 coined the term to mean "the analysis of

BOX 3-6
Case Study of Bone Mineral Density Loss During Space Missions

Space travel in low Earth orbit or beyond Earth's orbit exposes individuals (astronauts or cosmonauts) to environmental stresses (e.g., microgravity and cosmic radiation) that, if unabated, could result in radiation-induced physiological damage or marked physiological adaptation (microgravity-induced shifts in calcium and bone metabolism) that could be deleterious or even fatal during space travel, on landing on another planet, or after the return to Earth. Based on the preceding discussion of statistical prediction, one can consider the details of design and analysis of a potential study of bone mineral density loss in astronauts.

Assume that there are n control astronauts in either a simulated environment or on the International Space Station not taking part in a countermeasure program, or perhaps serving as matched control astronauts on Earth and n_i experimental subjects (e.g., astronauts subjected to experimental countermeasures) in each of p space missions. Let s_i be the number of subjects required to be contained within the interval for space mission i. For example, if n_i is equal to 5 and one wishes to have the median value in space mission i below the upper prediction limit, then s_i is equal to 3. An effect of the experimental intervention on a particular outcome measure is declared only if the s_ith largest measurement (e.g., the median) lies outside of the prediction interval (or above [below] the prediction limit in the one-sided case) in all p space missions. Statistical details for both parametric and nonparametric solutions to this problem are presented in Appendix A.

Returning to the example, suppose that a series of 20 control astronauts on Earth are monitored for the same period of time that 5 astronauts on a single space mission are evaluated for the effects of a series of countermeasures on bone mineral density loss. The question is whether the countermeasures are sufficient to eliminate the effect of the space mission on bone mineral density loss, such that the bone mineral density measurements for the experimental astronauts are consistent with the bone mineral density measurements for the control astronauts. To this end, consider a comparison of the maximum of 20 control measurements ($n = u = 20$) with the median for a single space mission ($p = 1$) with n_i equal to five experimental astronauts (i.e., $s_i = 3$) for a single outcome measure (Case A). Using the previous equations, one obtains an overall confidence level of 99.6 percent, indicating an extremely low probability that the experimental median will be above the largest control bone mineral density measurement by chance alone. One can do better, however. Instead of selecting the most extreme control measurement, take the 18th largest measurement (Case B). In this case, the confidence is 96 percent and one has a more powerful decision rule. Now, consider the effects of multiple endpoints (Case C). With k equal to 10 endpoints and the prediction limit defined as the 18th largest control measurement, the overall confidence level for the experiment is reduced to 68 percent. To counteract this effect (Case D), one can add a second space mission ($p = 2$), each with n_i equal to five astronauts, and the overall confidence is increased back to 96 percent. If one had instead considered p equal to four space missions (Case E), a confidence of 94 percent would be achieved by setting the prediction limit to the 15th largest control measurement, again increasing the statistical power of the decision rule.

How does one select from among the various strategies described in the simple example described above? The answer is to select the strategy that has reasonable confidence (i.e., a low rate of false-positive results, e.g., 5 percent) and that has the maximum statistical power for a desired effect size. To this end, one can evaluate the power of the test to detect a true difference between the control group and the experimental group by simulation.

analyses." Meta-analysis is widely used in education (see Box 3-7), psychology, and the medical sciences (e.g., in evidence-based medicine) and has frequently been used to study the efficacies of different treatments (Hedges and Olkin, 1985).

A meta-analysis can summarize an entire set of research in the literature, a sample from a large population of studies, or some defined subset of studies (e.g., published studies or *n*-of-1 studies). The degree to which the results of a synthesis can be generalized depends in part on the nature of the set of studies. In general, meta-analysis serves as a useful tool to answer questions for which single trials were underpowered or not designed to address. More specifically, the following are benefits of meta-analysis:

- It can provide a way to combine the results of studies with different designs (within reason) when similar research questions are of interest.
- It uses a common outcome metric when studies vary in the ways in which outcomes are measured.
- It accounts for differences in precision, typically by weighting in proportion to sample size.
- Its indices are based on sufficient statistics.
- It can examine between-study differences in results (heterogeneity).

It can examine the relationship of study outcomes to study features (Becker, 2000).

TABLE 3-2 Key Points in the Conduct of Meta-Analyses

- Systematic reviews of study findings often use complex statistical methods to synthesize and interpret data from individual studies, and an understanding of their basic principles is important in interpreting their results.
- Quantitative synthesis cannot replace sound clinical reasoning; combining poor-quality or overly biased data that do not make sense is likely to produce unreliable results.
- When appropriate, combining data from various studies to obtain a common estimate can increase the statistical power for the discovery of treatment efficacy and can increase the precision of the estimate.
- Sensitivity analyses should be performed to determine the robustness of conclusions.
- Patients, clinical settings, and treatment responses are expected to vary across trials that have studied the same problem. Insight into reasons for the heterogeneity of trial results may often be as important as or even more important than producing aggregate results.

SOURCE: Lau, Ioannidis, and Schmid (1997).

BOX 3-7
Combining *n*-of-1 Studies in Meta-Analysis: Results from Research in Special Education

Researchers in special education are often concerned with individualized treatments for behavior disorders or with low-incidence disabilities and disorders. Single-case research designs are quite common. Study designs typically involve a baseline period followed by a treatment period and possibly follow-up. Multiple measures are usually obtained from each case during the baseline and treatment. Crossover treatment designs are occasionally used and usually involve only two baseline-treatment cycles. Meta-analysis has been applied since the 1980s to summarize these case-study designs.

However, the methods proposed have been controversial and the statistical properties of the methods have not been rigorously studied. Three approaches have been used to measure effects.

(1) ***Single-case effect size.*** Some researchers have used an index similar to the effect size, computed for $n > 1$ studies as the standardized difference between group means:

$$g = \frac{\overline{Y}_{treatment} - \overline{Y}_{baseline}}{S_{y\,pooled}}$$

$\overline{Y}_{treatment}$ is the subject's mean score during treatment, $\overline{Y}_{baseline}$ is the mean before treatment, and $S_{Y\,pooled}$ is obtained by pooling intrasubject variation across the two time periods.

(2) ***Percentage of nonoverlapping data index (PND)*** (Scruggs, Mastropieri, and Castro, 1987). The percentage of nonoverlapping data index is also based on the idea of examining the data from the baseline and treatment periods of the case study. The index is the percentage of datum values observed during treatment that exceed the highest baseline data value.

(3) ***Regression approaches*** (Center, Skiba, and Casey, 1986). The researcher estimates the treatment effect and separate effects of time during baseline ($t = 1$ to n_a) and treatment ($t = n_a$ to n) phases via

$$Y_i = b_0 + b_1 X_i + b_2 t + b_3 X_i (t - n_a) + e_i$$

The effects of interest, say, b_1 for X or b_3 for $X(t)$, are then evaluated via incremental F tests, which are transformed and summarized.

A relevant question is: when does a meta-analysis of small studies rule out the need for a large trial? One investigation showed that the results of smaller trials are usually compatible with the results of larger trials, although large studies may produce a more precise answer to a particular question when the treatment effect is not large but is clinically important (Cappelleri, Ioannidis, Schmid, et al., 1996). When the small studies are replicates of each other—as, for example, in collaborative laboratory or clinical studies or when there has been a concerted effort to corroborate a single small study that has produced an unexpected result—a meta-analysis may be conclusive if the combined statistical power is sufficient. Even when small studies are replicates of one another, however, the population to which they refer may be very narrow. In addition, when the small studies differ too much, the populations may be too broad to be of much use (Flournoy and Olkin, 1995). Some have suggested that the use of meta-analysis to predict the results of future studies is important but would require a design format not currently used (Flournoy and Olkin, 1995).

Meta-analysis involves the designation of an effect size and a method of analysis. In the case of proportions, some of the effect sizes used are risk differences, risk ratios, odds ratios, number needed to treat, variance-stabilized risk differences, and differences between expected and observed outcomes. For continuous outcomes, the standardized mean difference or correlations are common measures. The technical aspects of these procedures have been developed by Hedges and Olkin (1985).

Meta-analysis sometimes refers to the entire process of synthesizing the results of independent studies, including the collection of studies, coding, abstracting, and so on, as well as the statistical analysis. However, some researchers use the term to refer to only the statistical portion, which includes methods such as the analysis of variance, regression, Bayesian analysis and multivariate analysis. The confidence profile method (CPM), another form of meta-analysis (Eddy, Hasselblad, and Shacter, 1992) adopts the first definition of meta-analysis and attempts to deal with all the issues in the process, such as alternative designs, outcomes, and biases, as well as the statistical analysis, which is Bayesian. Methods of analysis used for CPM include analysis of variance, regression, nonparametric analysis, and Bayesian analysis. The CPM analysis approach differs from other meta-analysis techniques based on classical statistics in that it provides marginal probability distributions for the parameters of interest and if an integrated approach is used, a joint probability distribution for all the parameters. More common meta-analysis procedures provide a point estimate for one or more effect sizes together with confidence intervals for the estimates. Although exact confidence intervals can be obtained using numerical integration, large sample approximations often provide sufficiently accurate results even when the sample sizes are small.

Some have suggested that those who use meta-analysis should go beyond the point estimates and confidence intervals that represent the aggregate findings of a meta-analysis and look carefully at the studies that were included to evaluate the consistency of their results. When the results are largely on the same side of the "no-difference" line, one may have more confidence in the results of a meta-analysis (LeLorier, Gregoire, Benhaddad, et al., 1997).

Sometimes small studies (including *n*-of-1 studies) are omitted from meta-analyses (Sandborn, McLeod, and Jewell, 1999). Others, however, view meta-analysis as a remedy or as a means to increase power relative to the power of individual small studies in a research domain (Kleiber and Harper, 1999). Because those who perform meta-analyses typically weight the results in proportion to sample size, small sample sizes have less of an effect on the results than larger ones. A synthesis based mainly on small sample sizes will produce summary results with more uncertainty (larger standard errors and wider confidence intervals) than a synthesis based on studies with larger sample sizes. Thus, a cumulative meta-analysis requires a stopping procedure that allows one to say that a treatment is or is not effective (Olkin, 1996).

When the combined trials are a homogeneous set designed to answer the same question for the same population, the use of a fixed-effects model, in which the estimated treatment effects vary across studies only as a result of random error, is appropriate (Lau, Ioannidis, and Schmid, 1998). To assess homogeneity, heterogeneity is often tested on the basis of the chi-square distribution, although this lacks power. If heterogeneity is detected, the traditional approach is to abort the meta-analysis or to use random-effects models. Random-effects models assume that no single treatment effect exists, but each study has a different true effect, with all treatment effects derived from a population of such truths assumed to follow a normal distribution (Lau, Ioannidis, and Schmid, 1998) (see section on Hiearchical Models and Appendix A). Neither fixed-effects nor random-effects models are entirely satisfactory because they either oversimplify or fail to explain heterogeneity. Meta-regressions of effect sizes affected by control rates have been used to develop reasons for observed heterogeneity and to attempt to identify significant relations between the treatment effect and the covariates of interest; however, a significant association in regression analysis does not prove causality. Because heterogeneity can be a problem in the interpretation of a meta-analysis, an empirical study (Engels, Terrin, Barza, et al., 2000) showed that, in general, random-effects models for odds ratios and risk differences yielded similar results. The same was true for fixed-effects models. Random-effects models were more conservative both for risk differences and for odds ratios. When studies are homogeneous it appears that there is consistency of results when risk differences or odds ratios are used and consistency of results when random-effects or fixed-effects models are used. Differences appear when heterogeneity is present (Engels, Terrin, Barza, et al., 2000).

The use of an individual subject's data rather than summary data from each study can circumvent ecological fallacies. Such analyses can provide maximum information about covariates to which heterogeneity can be ascribed and allow for a time-to-event analysis (Lau, Ioannidis, and Schmid, 1998). Like large-scale clinical trials, meta-analyses cannot always show how individuals should be treated, even if they are useful for estimation of a population effect. Patients may respond differently to a treatment. To address this diversity, meta-analysis can rely on response-surface models to summarize evidence along multiple covariates of interest. A reliable meta-analysis requires consistent, high-quality reporting of the primary data from individual studies.

Meta-analysis is a retrospective analytical method, the results of which will be based primarily on the rigor of the technique (the trial designs) and the quality of the trials being pooled. Cumulative meta-analysis can help determine when additional studies are needed and can improve the predictability of previous small trials (Villar, Carroli, and Belizan, 1995). Several workshops have produced a set of guidelines for the reporting of meta-analysis of randomized clinical trials (the Quality of Reporting of Meta-Analysis group statement [Moher, Cook, Eastwood, et al., 1999], the Consolidated Standard of Reporting Trials conference statement [Begg, Cho, Eastwood, et al., 1996], and the Meta-Analysis of Observational Studies in Epidemiology group statement on meta-analysis of observational studies [Stroup, Berlin, Morton, et al., 2000]).

RISK-BASED ALLOCATION

Empirical Bayes methods are needed for analysis of experiments with risk-based allocation for two reasons. First, the natural heterogeneity from subject to subject requires some accounting for random effects; and second, the differential selection of groups due to the risk-based allocation is handled perfectly by the "*u-v*" method introduced by Herbert E. Robbins. The *u*-v method of estimation capitalizes on certain general properties of distributions such as the Poisson or normal distribution that hold under arbitrary and unknown mixtures of parameters, thus allowing for the existence of random effects. At the same time, the *u-v* method allows estimation of averages under a wide family of restrictions on the sample space, such as restriction to high-risk or low-risk subjects, thus addressing the risk-based allocation design feature. These ideas and approaches are considered in greater detail in Appendix A.

Another example from Finkelstein, Levin, and Robbins (1996b) given in Box 3-8 illustrates the application of risk-based allocation to a trial studying the occurrence of opportunistic infections in very sick AIDS patients. This example was taken from an actual randomized trial, ACTG Protocol 002, which tested the efficacy of low-dose versus high-dose zidovudine (AZT). Survival time was the primary endpoint of the clinical trial, but for the purpose of illustrating risk-based allocation, Finkelstein and colleagues focused on the secondary endpoint of opportunistic infections. They studied the rate of such infections per year of follow-up time with an experimental low dose of AZT that they hoped was better tolerated by patients and which would thereby improve the therapeutic efficacy of the treatment.

SUMMARY

Because the choice of a study design for a small clinical trial is constrained by size, the power and effectiveness of such studies may be diminished, but these need not be completely lost. Small clinical trials frequently need to be viewed as part of a process of continuing data collection; thus, the objectives of a small clinical trial should be understood in that context. For example, a small clinical trial often guides the design of a subsequent trial. Therefore, a key question will be what information from the current trial will be of greatest value in designing the next one? In small clinical trials of drugs, for example, the most important result might be to provide information on the type of postmarketing surveillance that should follow.

A major fundamental question is the qualitatively different goals that one might have when studying very few people. The main example here is determination of the best treatment that allows astronauts to avoid bone mineral density loss. Such research could have many goals. One goal would be to provide information on this phenomenon that is most likely to be correct in some universal sense; that is, the knowledge and estimates are as unbiased and as precise as possible. A second goal might be to treat the most astronauts in the manner that was most likely to be optimal for each individual. These are profoundly different goals that would have to be both articulated and discussed before any trial designs could be considered. One can find the components of a goal discussion in some of the descriptions of individual designs, but the discussion of goals is not identified as part of a

BOX 3-8
Illustration of a Clinical Trial on Opportunistic Infections Using Risk-Based Allocation Analysis

A total of 512 subjects were randomly assigned in ACTG Protocol 002 to evaluate the therapeutic efficacy of an experimental low dose of AZT (500 mg/day) versus the high dose of AZT (1,500 mg/day) that was the standard dose at the time of the trial. A total of 254 patients were randomized to the low-dose experimental group and 258 were randomized to the high-dose standard treatment group. Although all patients in the original trial were seriously immunodeficient, the focus here is on the treatment effect among the subgroup of 253 patients at highest risk, defined as those with initial CD4-cell counts less than or equal to 60 per microliter of blood. In this subgroup, the number of opportunistic infections among the 125 patients in the high-dose (standard) treatment group was observed to be 296 with 66,186 days of follow-up, for an opportunistic infection rate of 1.632 per year. Among the 128 high-risk patients randomized to the low-dose (experimental) treatment group, the number of opportunistic infections was 262 with 75,591 days of follow-up, for an opportunistic infection rate of 1.265 per year. The ratio of the rate for the control group to the treatment group is 1.632/1.265 = 1.290, with a standard error of ±0.109. Thus, the "gold standard" (randomized) estimate of the low-dose effect on the high-risk patients is that it reduces their rate of opportunistic infections by about 22.5 percent (1−1/1.290 = 0.225) relative to that for the higher-dose group.

If the trial had used risk-based allocation with all of the high-risk patients receiving the experimental low dose and all of the lower-risk patients (with CD4-cell counts >60 per microliter) receiving the standard high dose, the effect of the standard dose on the high-risk patients would have been estimated instead of being directly observed. This is done by first fitting a model for the rate of opportunistic infections under standard treatment with the data for the lower-risk patients. Previous data suggest that the annual rate of opportunistic infection under the standard dose can be modeled by the exponential function $R(X) = A\ exp\ (BX)$, where X is the CD4-cell count per microliter at the start of the trial, and A and B are constants to be estimated from the trial data for the lower-risk patients. The rate $R(X)$ is the expected number of opportunistic infections per year of survival per patient for those with initial CD4-cell count X. A Poisson regression model was used, which assumes that the number of opportunistic infections occurring in a given time period t under standard treatment has a Poisson distribution with mean $tR(X)$. By using the data for the 133 lower-risk patients who received the standard dose, the maximum-likelihood estimates of the model parameters are $A = 0.541$ and $B = -0.00155$. The model estimates that with a CD4-cell count of, for example, 60 per microliter, the opportunistic infection rate would be 1.452 per year, whereas with a CD4-cell count of 10 per microliter it would be 1.526 per year. The total expected number of opportunistic infections for the high-risk patients under standard treatment is the sum of the model expectations over all 128 high-risk patients (who in fact received the low dose). That sum is 340.46, whereas the actual number is 262. The estimated rate ratio among the high-risk patients is thus 340.46/262 = 1.2995 (with a standard error of approximately ±0.147 after adjusting for overdispersion). Under risk-based allocation, then, the estimated low-dose effect on the high-risk patients is a reduction in the rate of opportunistic infection of 23.0 percent (1 − 1/1.2995 = 0.230), close to the randomized estimate of 22.5 percent. In the estimation of the rate ratio, the use of risk-based allocation and an appropriate model generated results that are virtually indistinguishable from those generated by the randomized clinical trial.

SOURCE: Finkelstein, Levin, and Robbins (1996b).

conceptual framework that would go into choosing which class of trials to be used.

It is quite likely that there could be very substantial disagreement about those goals. The first might lead one to include every subject in a defined time period (e.g., 10 missions) in one grand experimental protocol. The second might lead one to identify a subgroup of individuals who would be the initial experimental subjects and whose results would be applied to the remainder of the subjects. On the other hand, it might lead to a series of intensive metabolic studies for each individual, including, perhaps, *n*-of-1 type trials, which might be best for the individualization of therapy but not for the production of generalizable knowledge.

Situations may arise in which it is impossible to answer a question with any confidence. In those cases, the best that one can do is use the information to develop new research questions. In other cases, it may be necessary to answer the question as best as possible because a major, possibly irreversible decision must be made. In those cases, multiple, corroborative analyses might boost confidence in the findings.

RECOMMENDATIONS

Early consideration of possible statistical analyses should be an integral part of the study design. Once the data are collected, alternative statistical analyses should be used to bolster confidence in the interpretation of results. For example, if one is performing a Bayesian analysis, a non-Bayesian analysis should also be performed, and vice versa; similar cross-validation of other techniques should also be considered.

> **RECOMMENDATION: Perform corroborative statistical analyses. Given the greater uncertainties inherent in small clinical trials, several alternative statistical analyses should be performed to evaluate the consistency and robustness of the results of a small clinical trial.**

The use of alternative statistical analyses might help identify the more sensitive variables and the key interactions in applying heterogeneous results across trials or in trying to make generalizations across trials. In small clinical trials, more so than in large clinical trials, one must be particularly cautious about recognizing individual variability among subjects in terms of their biology and health care preferences, and administrative variability in terms of what can be done from one setting to another. The diminished power of studies with small sample sizes might mean that the generalizability of the findings might not be a possibility in the short-term, if at all. Thus, caution should be exercised in the interpretation of the results from small clinical trials.

RECOMMENDATION: Exercise caution in interpretation. One should exercise caution in the interpretation of the results of small clinical trials before attempting to extrapolate or generalize those results.

4
General Guidelines

This report has surveyed a large number of experimental design and analysis strategies that are useful, at least to some degree, in studies with small numbers of participants. Throughout the report the committee has pointed out that, whenever possible, large and adequately powered randomized clinical trials are the method of choice. The committee has also noted that in some cases such studies are impractical or impossible to conduct and that one must derive inferences from less rigorously controlled studies with less statistical power. To this end, the committee has presented several different designs that can be used in a variety of different circumstances in which full randomized clinical trials are not possible. In addition, the committee has presented several different analytical strategies, some common and others somewhat novel, that form a basic toolkit for small clinical studies. Here the committee provides some basic guidance on types of trial designs and analysis strategies that should be used and the circumstances in which they should be used. The reader should note that this guidance is limited, and different approaches or combinations of these approaches may be more useful in a specific setting.

The committee has discussed a variety of analysis issues, including sequential analysis, hierarchical models, Bayesian analysis, decision analysis, statistical prediction, meta-analysis, and risk-based allocation. When an investigator is attempting to better understand a dose-response relation or a response surface and has limited resources, sequential analysis is an ideal technique. It allows an adaptive approach to the allocation of resources in the most efficient way possible, such that one may identify an optimal dosage or set of conditions with the smallest number of participants.

When the data are collected in clusters, for example, from space missions or through collaboration with several clinics, hierarchical models, meta-analysis, or statistical prediction strategies may be useful. When choosing among these, consider the following. Meta-analysis can be used if different outcome or assessment measures are used for the different clusters such that each cluster is a separate study. The advantage of meta-analysis is that it allows one to combine information from studies or cluster samples that do not share a common endpoint. By contrast, a hierarchical model can be used if the studies or clusters contain both experimental and control conditions and they all use the same endpoint. The hierarchical model will adjust the standard errors of the estimated parameters for the within-cluster correlation that is produced by sharing a common environment. Hierarchical models are also the method of choice when there are repeated measurements for the same individuals, either over time or in a crossover study in which each participant is subjected to two or more treatment conditions. In this case the individual is the cluster and the hierarchical model is a method that can be used to put together what are essentially a series of *n*-of-1 experiments with a sample size of 1 (*n*-of 1 experiments). In some cases, however, each cluster may contain only experimental participants and one wishes to compare the clusters sequentially with a historical or parallel control group. Typically, the latter groups are larger. Since control and experimental conditions are not nested within clusters, hierarchical models do not apply and in fact would confound the difference between experimental measurements and the control measurements within the random cluster effect. This case is treated, however, as a problem of statistical prediction, in which the control measurements are used to derive an interval that will contain a proportion of the experimental measurements (e.g., 50 percent or the median) in each cluster with a reasonable level of confidence.

By contrast, decision analysis, Bayesian approaches, and ranking and selection are generally used to arrive at a decision about whether a particular intervention is useful or better than some alternative. These approaches are generally more subjective and may call for expert opinions to reach a final decision. Bayesian methods underlie many of the methods described here, including prediction, meta-analysis, and hierarchical models. Among these, ranking and selection allow one to arrive at a statistically optimal solution with a modicum of subjective inputs; however, decision analysis often allows a more complete characterization of a problem. Coupled with Bayesian methods, decision analysis has the additional benefit of being able to assess the sensitivity of the decision rule to various inputs or assumptions that went into constructing the decision rule.

Finally, the committee has also presented risk-based allocation as a useful tool for research with small numbers of participants. This method is quite different from the others but can be useful for those cases in which it may be unethical to withhold treatment from a high-risk population by randomly assigning them to a control group.

References

Alderson, P. 1996. Equipoise as a means of managing uncertainty: personal, communal and proxy. *Journal of Medical Ethics* 22:135–139.

Altman, L. K. 1996. Safety of catheter into the heart is questioned, startling doctors. *The New York Times*, September 18, p. A1.

Altman, L. K. 2000. Ethical and patient information concerns: who goes first? Presentation to the Institute of Medicine Committee on Strategies for Small-Number-Participant Clinical Research Trials, September 28, Washington, D.C.

Armitage, P. 1975. *Sequential Medical Trials.* New York: Wiley & Sons.

Becker, B. J. 2000. Meta-analysis of small *n* clinical trials. Presentation to the Institute of Medicine Committee on Strategies for Small-Number-Participant Clinical Research Trials, September 28, Washington, D.C.

Begg, C., M. Cho, S. Eastwood, R. Horton, D. Moher, I. Olkin, R. Pitkin, D. Rennie, K. Schulz, D. Simel, and D. Stroup. 1996. Improving the quality of reporting of randomized controlled trials: The CONSORT Statement. *Journal of the American Medical Association* 276:637–639.

Bhaumik, D. K., and R. D. Gibbons. An upper prediction limit for the arithmetic mean of a lognormal random variable. Submitted for publication.

Bock, R. D. 1979. Univariate and multivariate analysis of time-structured data. In: *Longitudinal Research in the Study of Behavior and Development.* J. R. Nesselroade and P. B. Baltes, eds. New York: Academic Press.

Bock, R. D. 1983. The discrete Bayesian. In: *Principles of Modern Psychological Measurement.* H. Wainer and S. Messick, eds. Hillsdale, NJ: Earlbaum.

Bock, R. D., ed. 1989. *Multilevel Analysis of Educational Data.* New York: Academic Press.

Boers, M., P. Brooks, V. Strand, and P. Tugwell. 1998. The OMERACT Filter for Outcome Measures in Rheumatology. *Journal of Rheumatology* 25:198–199.

Boers, M., P. Brooks, V. Strand, and P. Tugwell. 1999. OMERACT IV: Introduction. Fourth International Consensus Conference on Outcome Measures in Rheumatology. *Journal of Rheumatology* 26:199–200.

Brody, J. 1997. Alzheimer studies thwarted. *The New York Times*, March 5, p. C10.

Bryk, A. S., and S. W. Raudenbush. 1987. Application of hierarchical linear models to assessing change. *Psychological Bulletin* 101:47–158.

Bryk, A. S., and S. W. Raudenbush. 1992. *Hierarchical Linear Models: Applications and Data Analysis Methods*. Newbury Park, CA: Sage Publications.

Cappelleri, J. C., J. P. Ioannidis, C. H. Schmid, S. D. de Ferranti, M. Aubert, T. C. Chalmers, and J. Lau. 1996. Large trials vs meta-analysis of smaller trials: how do their results compare? *Journal of the American Medical Association* 276:1332–1338.

Center, B. A., R. J. Skiba, and A. Casey 1986. A methodology for the quantitative synthesis of intra-subject design research. *Journal of Special Education* 19:387–400.

Chi, E. M., and G. C. Reinsel. 1989. Models of longitudinal data with random effects and AR(1) errors. *Journal of the American Statistical Association* 84:452–459.

Chou, Y., and D. Owen. 1986. One-sided distribution-free simultaneous prediction limits for *p* future samples. *Journal of Quality Technology* 18:96–98.

Clark, P. I., and P. E. Leaverton. 1994. Scientific and ethical issues in the use of placebo controls in clinical trials. *Annual Review of Public Health* 15:19–38.

Cochran, W. G. 1968. The effectiveness of adjustment by subclassification in removing bias in observational studies. *Biometrics* 24:295–313.

Cox, D. R., and D. V. Hinkley. 1974. *Theoretical Statistics*. London: Chapman & Hall.

Davis, C. B. 1993. Environmental regulatory statistics. In: *Handbook of Statistics. Environmental Statistics, Vol. 12*. C. R. Rao, N. K. Bose, G. S. Maddala, H. D. Vinod, and G. P. Patil, eds. Amsterdam: North-Holland.

Davis, C. B., and R. J. McNichols. 1987. One-sided intervals for at least *p* of *m* observations from a normal population on each of *r* future occasions. *Technometrics* 29:359–370.

Day, S. J., and D. G. Altman. 2000. Blinding in clinical trials and other studies. *British Medical Journal* 321:504.

Delaney, M. 2000. Small clinical trials: tool or folly? Presentation to the Institute of Medicine Committee on Strategies for Small-Number-Participant Clinical Research Trials, September 28, Washington, D.C.

DeLeeuw, J., and I. Kreft. 1986. Random coefficient models for multilevel analysis. *Journal of Educational Statistics* 11:57–85.

Dempster, A. P., D. B. Rubin, and R. K. Tsutakawa. 1981. Estimation in covariance component models. *Journal of the American Statistical Society* 76:341–353.

Diggle, P., K. Y. Liang, and S. L. Zeger. 1994. *Analysis of Longitudinal Data*. New York: Oxford University Press.

Dixon, W. J., and A. M. Mood. 1948. A method for obtaining and analyzing sensitivity data. *Journal of the American Statistical Association* 43:109–126.

Dodge, H. F., and H. G. Romig. 1929. A method for sampling inspection. *Bell System Technical Journal* 8:613–631.

Drummond, M. F., B. O'Brien, G. L. Stoddart, and G. W. Torrance. 1997. *Methods for the Economic Evaluation of Health Care Programmes*, 2nd ed. Oxford: Oxford University Press.

Dunnett, C. W. 1955. A multiple comparisons procedure for comparing several treatments with a control. *Journal of the American Statistical Association* 50:1096–1121.

Durham, S., N. Flournoy, and W. F. Rosenberger. 1997. A random walk rule for phase I clinical trials. *Biometrics* 53:745–760.

Eddy, D. M., V. Hasselblad, and R. Shachter. 1992. *Meta-Analysis by the Confidence Profile Method. The Statistical Synthesis of Evidence.* San Diego: Academic Press.

Edgington, E. S. 1996. Randomized single-subject experimental designs. *Behaviour Research and Therapy* 34:567–574.

Elston, R. C., and J. E. Grizzle. 1962. Estimation of time-response curves and their confidence bands. *Biometrics* 18:148–159.

Emond, J. 2000. Progress in surgery: innovation or research? Presentation to the Institute of Medicine Committee on Strategies for Small-Number-Participant Clinical Research Trials, September 28, Washington, D.C.

Engels, E. A., N. Terrin, M. Barza, and J. Lau. 2000. Meta-analysis of diagnostic tests for acute sinusitis. *Journal of Clinical Epidemiology* 53:852–862.

Environmental Protection Agency. 1992. *Addendum to the Interim Final Guidance Document. Statistical Analysis of Ground-Water Monitoring Data at RCRA Facilities.* Washington, D.C.: Enviromental Protection Agency.

Farewell, V. T., and G. J. D'Angio. 1981. A simulated study of historical controls using real data. *Biometrics* 37:169–176.

Faustman, D. L. 2000. Small clinical research trials: needs beyond space. Presentation to the Institute of Medicine Committee on Strategies for Small-Number-Participant Clinical Research Trials, September 28, Washington, D.C.

Fearn, T. 1975. A Bayesian approach to growth curves. *Biometrika* 62:89–100.

Feiveson, A. H. 2000. Quantitative assessment of countermeasure efficacy for long-term space missions. Presentation to the Institute of Medicine Committee on Strategies for Small-Number- Participant Clinical Research Trials, September 28, Washington, D.C.

Finkelstein, M. O., and B. Levin. 1990. *Statisics for Lawyers.* New York: Springer-Verlag.

Finkelstein, M. O., B. Levin, and H. Robbins. 1996a. Clinical and prophylactic trials with assured new treatment for those at greater risk. Part I. Introduction. *American Journal of Public Health* 86:691–695.

Finkelstein, M. O., B. Levin, and H. Robbins. 1996b. Clinical and prophylactic trials with assured new treatment for those at greater risk. Part II. Examples. *American Journal of Public Health* 86:696–705.

Fisher, R. A. 1935. *The Design of Experiments.* Edinburgh: Oliver and Boyd.

Flournoy, N. (in press). Up-and-down designs. In: *Encyclopedia of Envirometrics.* London: Wiley.

Flournoy, N., and I. Olkin. 1995. Do small trials square with large ones? *Lancet* 345:741–742.

Food and Drug Administration. 1999. International Conference on Harmonisation; E10 Choice of control group in clinical trials: draft guidance. *Federal Register* 64:51767–51780.

Freedman, B. 1987. Equipoise and the ethics of clinical research. *New England Journal of Medicine* 317:141–145.

Friedman, L. M., C. D. Furberg, and D. L. DeMets. 1996. *Fundamentals of Clinical Trials.* Boston: Wright.

Gehan, E. A. 1982. Design of controlled clinical trials: use of historical controls. *Cancer Treatment Reports* 66:1089–1093.

Gibbons, R. D. 1987a. Statistical models for the analysis of volatile organic compounds in waste disposal sites. *Ground Water* 25:572–580.

Gibbons, R. D. 1987b. Statistical prediction intervals for the evaluation of ground-water equality.

Ground Water 25:455–465.

Gibbons, R. D. 1990. A general statistical procedure for ground-water detection monitoring at waste disposal facilities. *Ground Water* 28:235–243.

Gibbons, R. D. 1991. Some additional nonparametric prediction limits for ground-water detection monitoring at waste disposal facilities. *Ground Water* 29:729–736.

Gibbons, R .D. 1994. *Statistical Methods for Groundwater Monitoring.* New York: Wiley.

Gibbons, R. D. 1996. Some conceptual and statistical issues in analysis of ground-water monitoring data. *Environmetrics* 7:185–199.

Gibbons, R. D. 2000. Mixed-effects models for mental health services research. *Health Services and Outcomes Research Methodology* 1:91–129.

Gibbons, J. D., I. Olkin, and M. Sobel. 1979. An introduction to ranking and selection. *The American Statistician* 33:185–192.

Gibbons, R. D., and D. Hedeker. 2000. Applications of mixed-effect models in biostatistics. *Sankhya* 62 Series B:70–103.

Gibbons, R. D., D. R. Cox, D. R. Grayson, D. K. Bhaumik, J. M. Davis, and R. P. Sharma. (under review). Sequential prediction bounds for identifying differentially expressed genes in replicated microarray experiments. *Biometrics.*

Goldstein, H. 1986. Multilevel mixed linear model analysis using iterative generalized least squares *Biometrika* 73:43–56.

Goldstein, H. 1995. *Multilevel Statistical Models*, 2nd ed. New York: Halstead Press.

Gow, P. J., and D. Mutimer. 2001. Liver transplantation for an HIV-positive patient in the era of highly active antiretroviral therapy. *AIDS* 26:291-292.

Guttman, I. 1970. *Statistical Tolerance Regions: Classical and Bayesian.* Darien, Conn: Hafner.

Guyatt, G. H. 1986. The treatment of heart failure. A methodological review of the literature. *Drugs* 32:538–568.

Guyatt, G. H., D. Sackett, J. Adachi, R. Roberts, J. Chong, D. Rosenbloom, and J. Keller. 1988. A clinician's guide for conducting randomized trials in individual patients. *Canadian Medical Association Journal* 139:497–503.

Hahn, G. J., and W. O. Meeker. 1991. *Statistical Intervals: A Guide for Practitioners.* New York: Wiley.

Harville, D. A. 1977. Maximum likelihood approaches to variance component estimation and to related problems. *Journal of the American Statistical Association* 72:320–385.

Hauck, W. W., and S. Anderson. 1999. Some issues in the design and analysis of equivalence trials. *Drug Information Journal* 33:109–118.

Hedayat, A. S., A. J. Izenman, and W. G. Zhang. 1996. Random sampling for forensic study of controlled substances, 12–21. In: *Proceedings of the Section on Physical and Engineering Sciences American Statistical Association.* Alexandria, VA: American Statistical Association.

Hedeker, D. R., R. D. Gibbons, and C. Waternaux. 1999. Sample size estimation for longitudinal designs with attrition. *Journal of Educational Statistics* 24:70–93.

Hedges, L. V., and I. Olkin. 1985. Introduction. In: *Statistical Methods for Meta-Analysis*. I. Olkin and L. V. Hedges, eds. New York: Academic Press.

Heitjan, D. F. 1997. Bayesian interim analysis of phase II cancer clinical trials. *Statistics in Medicine* 16:1791–1802.

Heyd, J. M., and B. P. Carlin. 1999. Adaptive design improvements in the continual reassessment method for phase I studies. *Statistics in Medicine* 18:1307–1321.

Hillner, B. E., and R. M. Centor. 1987. What a difference a day makes: a decision analysis of adult streptococcal pharyngitis. *Journal of General Internal Medicine* 2:244–250.

Hoel, D. G., M. Sobel, and G. Weiss. 1975. A survey of adaptive sampling for clinical trials. In: *Perspectives in Biometrics*. R. M. Elashoff, ed. New York: Academic Press.

Hsieh, F. Y. 1988. Sample size formulae for intervention studies with the cluster as unit of randomization. *Statistics in Medicine* 8:1195–1201.

Institute of Medicine. 1992. *Medical Intervention at the Crossroads: Modern Methods of Clinical Investigation*. Washington, DC: National Academy Press.

James, W., and C. Stein. 1961. Estimation with quadratic loss. In: *Proceedings of the Berkeley Symposium on Mathematical Statistics and Probability*. J. Neyman, ed. Berkeley: University of California Press.

Jennison, C. and B. W. Turnbull. 1983. Confidence intervals for a binomial parameter following a multistage test with application to MIL-STD 105D and medical trials. *Technometrics* 25:49–58.

Johannessen, T. 1991. Controlled trials in single subjects. 1. Value in clinical medicine. *British Medical Journal* 303:173–174.

Jones, R. H. 1993. *Longitudinal Data Analysis with Serial Correlation: A State-Space Approach*. New York: Chapman & Hall.

Kim, K., and D. L. DeMets. 1992. Sample size determination for group sequential clinical trials with immediate response. *Statistics in Medicine* 11:1391–1399.

Kleiber, C., and D. C. Harper. 1999. Effects of distraction on children's pain and distress during medical procedures: a meta-analysis. *Nursing Research* 48:44–49.

Kolata, G. 1995. Women resist trials to test marrow transplants. *The New York Times*, February 15, p. C8.

Kolata, G. 1997. Lack of volunteers thwarts research on prostate cancer. *The New York Times*, February 12, p. A18.

Kolata, G., and K. Eichenwald. 1999. Business thrives on unproven care, leaving science behind. *The New York Times*, October 3, p. A1.

Kpamegan E. E., and N. Flournoy. 2001. An optimizing up-and-down design. In: *Optimum Design*. Boston: Kluwer.

Kraemer, H. C., and S. Thiemann. 1987. *How Many Subjects?: Statistical Power Analysis in Research*. New York: Sage Publications.

Krishnamurti, L., B. R. Blazar, and J. E. Wagner. 2001. Bone marrow transplantation without myeloablation for sickle cell disease. *New England Journal of Medicine* 344:68.

Lai, T. L., B. Levin, H. Robbins, and D. Siegmund. 1980. Sequential medical trials. *Proceedings of the National Academy of Sciences USA* 77:3135–3138.

Lai, T. L., and D. Siegmund, eds. 1985. *Herbert Robbins Selected Papers*. New York: Springer-Verlag.

Laird, N. M. and J. H. Ware. 1982. Random effects models for longitudinal data. *Biometrics* 38:963–974.

Lau, J., J. P. A. Ioannidis, and C. H. Schmid, 1997. Quantitative synthesis in systematic reviews. *Annals of Internal Medicine* 127:820–826.

Lau, J., J. P. A. Ioannidis, and C. H. Schmid. 1998. Summing up evidence: one answer is not always enough. *The Lancet* 351:123–127.

LeLorier, J., G. Gregoire, A. Benhaddad, J. Lapierre, and F. Derderian. 1997. Discrepancies between meta-analyses and subsequent large randomized, controlled trials. *New England Journal of Medicine* 337:536–542.

Levin, B., and H. Robbins. 1981. Selecting the highest probability in binomial or multinomial trials. *Proceedings of the National Academy of Sciences USA* 78:4663–4666.

Lilford, R. J., and J. Jackson. 1995. Equipoise and the ethics of randomization. *Journal of the Royal Society of Medicine* 88:552–559.

Lindley, D. V., and A. F. M. Smith. 1972. Bayes estimation for linear models. *Journal of the Royal Statistical Society Series B* 34:1–41.

Lindsey, J. K. 1993. *Models for Repeated Measurements.* New York: Oxford University Press.

Lipid Research Clinical Program. 1984. The Lipid Research Clinic's Coronary Primary Prevention Trial results. Parts I and II. *Journal of the American Medical Association* 251:354–374.

Longford, N. T. 1987. A fast scoring algorithm for maximum likelihood estimation in unbalanced mixed models with nested effects *Biometrika* 74:817–827.

Longford, N. T. 1993. *Random Coefficient Models.* New York: Oxford University Press.

Malakoff, D. 1999. Bayes offers a 'new' way to make sense of numbers. *Science* 286:1460–1464.

Mansour, H., E. V. Nordheim, and J. J. Rutledge. 1985. Maximum likelihood estimation of variance components in repeated measures designs assuming autoregressive errors. *Biometrics* 41:287–294.

Matthews, J. N. S. 1995. Small clinical trials: are they all bad? *Statistics in Medicine* 14:115–126.

Meinert, C. 1996. *Clinical Trials Dictionary: Terminology and Usage Recommendations.* Baltimore: Harbor Duvall Press.

Meinert, C. 2000. Future directions for small *n* clinical research trials. Presentation to the Institute of Medicine Committee on Strategies for Small-Number-Participant Clinical Research Trials, September 28, Washington, D.C.

Mishoe, H. O. 2000. Research needs in developing small *n* clinical trials. Presentation to the Institute of Medicine Committee on Small-Number-Participant Clinical Research Trials, September 28, Washington, D.C.

Moher, D., D. J. Cook, S. Eastwood, I. Olkin, D. Rennie, and D. F. Stroup. 1999. Improving the quality of reports of meta-analyses of randomised controlled trials: the QUORUM statement. *The Lancet* 354:1896–1900.

Olkin, I. 1996. Meta-analysis: current issues in research synthesis. *Statistics in Medicine* 5:1253–1257.

Pauker, S. G. 2000. Decision analysis and small clinical trials. Presentation to the Institute of Medicine Committee on Strategies for Small-Number-Participant Clinical Research Trials, September 28, Washington, D.C.

Piantadosi, S. 1997. *Clinical Trials: A Methodologic Perspective.* New York: Wiley.

Pocock, S. J. 1984. *Clinical Trials: A Practical Approach.* New York: Wiley.

Pocock, S. J. 1996. The role of external evidence in data monitoring of a clinical trial. *Statistics in Medicine* 15:1285–1293.

Robbins, H. 1956. An empirical Bayes approach to statistics. In: *Proceedings of the Third Berkeley Symposium on Mathematics and Statistical Probability 1954-1955.* J. Neyman, ed. Berkeley: University of California Press.

Robbins, H. 1977. Prediction and estimation for the compound Poisson distribution. *Proceedings of the National Academy of Sciences USA* 74:2670–2671.

Robbins, H. 1993. Comparing two treatments under biased allocation. *La Gazette des Sciences Mathematique du Quebec* 15:35–41.

Robbins, H., and C. H. Zhang. 1988. Estimating a treatment effect under biased sampling. *Proceedings of the National Academy of Sciences USA* 85:3670–3672.

Robbins, H., and C. H. Zhang. 1989. Estimating the superiority of a drug to a placebo when all and only those patients at risk are treated with the drug. *Proceedings of the National Academy of Sciences USA* 86:3003–3005.

Robbins, H., and C. H. Zhang. 1991. Estimating a multiplicative treatment effect under biased allocation. *Biometrika* 78:349–354.

Rosenbaum, P., and D. Rubin. 1983. The central role of the propensity score in observational studies for causal effects. *Biometrika* 70:41-55.

Rosenberg, B. 1973. Linear regression with randomly dispersed parameters. *Biometrika* 60:65–72.

Rosenberger, W. F. 1996. New directions in adaptive designs. *Statistical Science* 11:137–149.

Royall, R. 1997. *Statistical Evidence: A Likelihood Paradigm.* London: Chapman & Hall.

Royall, R. 2000. On the probability of observing misleading statistical evidence. *Journal of the American Statistical Association* 95:760–768 (discussion, pp. 768–780).

Sacks, H., T. C. Chalmers, and H. Smith. 1982. Randomized versus historical controls for clinical trials. *The American Journal of Medicine* 72: 233–240.

Sandborn, W. J., R. McLeod, and D. P. Jewell. 1999. Medical therapy for induction and maintenance and remission in pouchitis: systematic review. *Inflammatory Bowel Disease* 5:33–39.

Sarhan, A., and B. Greenberg. 1962. *Contributions to Order Statistic.* New York: Wiley.

Scruggs, T. E., M. A. Mastropieri, and G. Castro. 1987. The quantitative synthesis of single subject research: methodology and validation. *Remedial and Special Education* 8:24–33.

Senn, S. 1993. *Cross-Over Trials in Clinical Research.* New York: Wiley.

Siegel, J. P. 2000. Small *n* clinical trials in the regulatory setting. Presentation to the Institute of Medicine Committee on Strategies for Small-Number-Participant Clinical Research Trials, September 28, Washington, D.C.

Stroup, D. F., J. A. Berlin, S. C. Morton, I. Olkin, G. D. Williamson, D. Rennie, D. Moher, B. Becker, T. A. Sipe, and S. B. Thacker. 2000. Meta-analysis of observational studies in epidemilogy. A proposal for reporting. *Journal of the American Medical Association* 283:2008–2012.

Sutherland, H. J., E. M. Meslin, and J. E. Till. 1994. What's missing from current clinical trials guidelines? A framework for integrating ethics, science and community context. *Journal of Clinical Ethics* 5:297–303.

Temple, R. 1996. Problems in interpreting active control equivalence trials. *Accountability in Research* 4:267–275.

Thall, P. F. 2000. Bayesian strategies for small *n* clinical trials. Presentation to the Institute of Medicine Committee on Strategies for Small-Number-Participant Clinical Research Trials, September 28, Washington, D.C.

Thall, P. F., and K. T. Russell. 1998. A strategy for dose-finding and safety monitoring based on efficacy and adverse outcomes in phase I/II clinical trials. *Biometrics* 54:251–264.

Thall , P. F., and H. G. Sung. 1998. Some extensions and applications of a Bayesian strategy for monitoring multiple outcomes in clinical trials. *Statistics in Medicine* 17:1563–1580.

Thall, P. F., R. M. Simon, and E. H. Estey. 1995. Bayesian sequential monitoring designs for single-arm clinical trials with multiple outcomes. *Statistics in Medicine* 14:357–379.

Thall, P. F., R. M. Simon, and Y. Shen. 2000. Approximate Bayesian evaluation of multiple treatment effects. *Biometrics* 56:213–219.

Truog, R. 1992. Randomized controlled trials: lessons from ECMO. *Clinical Research* 40:519–527.

Tugwell, P. and C. Bombardier. 1982. A methodologic framework for developing and selecting endpoints in clinical trials. *Journal of Rheumatology* 9:758–762.

Vico, L., P. Collet, A. Guignandon, M. Lafage-Proust, T. Thomas, and M. Rehailia. 2000. Effects of long-term microgravity exposure on cancellous and cortical weight-bearing bones of cosmonauts. *The Lancet* 355:1607–1611.

Villar, J., G. Carroli, and J. M. Belizan. 1995. Predictability of meta-analyses of randomized controlled trials. *The Lancet* 345:772–776.

Ware, J. H. 1989. Investigating therapies of potentially great benefit: ECMO. *Statistical Science* 4:298–340.

Whitehead, J. 1992. Overrunning and underrunning in sequential clinical trials. *Controlled Clinical Trials* 13:106–121.

Whitehead, J. 1997. *The Design and Analysis of Sequential Clinical Trials.* New York: Wiley.

Whitehead, J. 1999. A unified theory for sequential clinical trials. *Statistics in Medicine* 18:2271–2286.

Whitehead, J. and H. Brunier, 1995. Bayesian decision procedures for dose determining experiments. *Statistics in Medicine* 14:885–893 (discussion, pp. 895–899).

World Medical Association. 1964. *Declaration of Helsinki. Adopted by the 18th World Medical Assembly Helsinki, Finland, and amended by the 29th World Medical Assembly Tokyo, Japan, 1975, the 35th World Medical Assembly Venice, Italy, 1983, and the 41st World Medical Assembly Hong Kong, 1989.* Edinburgh: World Medical Association.

World Medical Association. 2000. *Declaration of Helsinki: Ethical Principles for Medical Research Involving Human Subjects* (5th rev). Edinburgh: World Medical Association.

Zelen, M. 1969. Play the winner rule and the controlled clinical trial. *Journal of the American Statistical Association* 64:131–146.

Zivin, J. A. 2000. Understanding clinical trials. *Scientific American* 282:69–75.

Zucker, D. 2000. N-of-1 trials and combining N-of-1 trials to assess treatment effectiveness. Presentation to the Institute of Medicine Committee on Strategies for Small-Number-Participant Clinical Research Trials, September 28, Washington, D.C.

Zucker, D. R., C. H. Schmid, M. W. McIntosh, R. B. D'Agostino, H. P. Selker, and J. Lau. 1997. Combining single patient trials to estimate population treatment effects and to evaluate individual patient responses to treatment. *Journal of Clinical Epidemiology* 50:401–410.

Appendixes

Appendix A
Study Methods

STRATEGIES FOR GATHERING INFORMATION

Traditional Literature Searches

Electronic Data Bases

The initial step in developing an evidence-based research base for the study described in this report was a targeted search of the National Library of Medicine's Medline. The basic subject search terms included *Bayesian*, *sequential analysis*, *decision analysis*, *meta-analysis*, and *confidence profile method*. These are the methods of analysis that the committee had been charged with assessing as they relate to the conduct of clinical trials with small sample sizes. The search also used a combination of each subject search term with descriptors such as *models*, *statistical*, *clinical trials* or *randomized clinical trials*, *phase I*, *phase II*, *phase III*, *small sample*, and *n-of-1*. For example, one set of subject search terms is "models, statistical[mh] AND sequential analysis AND ("clinical trials" OR "randomized clinical trials")[mh] AND phase I." (MeSH is the abbreviation for medical subject heading. [mh] is used as a tag to tell the search engine to look for the terms in the MeSH fields of the Medline database.) Abstracts from the initial search were reviewed for relevance to the committee's charge and the more prominent authors (defined by having published at least 10 articles) were determined. Then a search by author name was done. A greater part of Appendix C, Selected Bibliography on Statistical and Small Clinical Trials Research, was the result of literature searches from the Medline database.

Databases such as Mathsci, Scisearch, and Pascal were used to verify the bibliographic information in the statistics literature that Medline does not cover. The Library of Congress Online Catalog and Social SciSearch were also searched for specific titles and authors provided by committee members.

Clinical Trials Listserv

A posting in a clinical trials *listserv* (clinical-trial@listserv.acor.org) that requested literature on small-number clinical trials generated several suggestions from all over the United States and a few from other countries. Their abstracts were obtained from Medline and reviewed for relevance to the study. Several suggestions that originated from responses to this *listserv* posting are included in Appendix C.

Other Sources

Special attention was given to references included in benchmark publications on the subject of small-number clinical trials. Abstracts of these references were also obtained from Medline. Several of these references are included in Appendix C. Additionally, valuable suggestions for relevant literature came from statisticians in other units of The National Academies and the Washington, D.C. academic community. Their suggestions are also included in Appendix C.

Selections by Committee Members

The preliminary list of background literature was circulated to the committee members. During the first committee conference call, committee members agreed to identify and submit to Institute of Medicine staff references (included or not included in the preliminary list) that they believe should be reviewed by the entire committee. The committee members' selections were then compiled, and copies were included in the first committee meeting briefing book for study by the committee members. Additionally, through the duration of the project, other published literature and unpublished data that committee members believed should be reviewed by the entire committee were obtained and circulated to the committee. Literature selections from committee members are added in Appendix C. Literature reviewed by the entire committee and used to prepare this report are cited in the References section.

One-Day Invitational Conference

In fulfilling the second task of the committee, a 1-day conference was convened on September 28, 2000, in Washington, D.C. More than 200 professionals from federal research and regulatory agencies, academia, industry, and other areas of clinical research and health care practice were invited to participate. The conference focused on the state of the science, challenges, and strategies in the design and evaluation of clinical trials of drugs, biologics, devices, and other medical interventions with populations with small numbers of individuals. Methods including randomized clinical trials, sequential clinical trials, meta-analysis, and decision analysis were considered in terms of their potentials and their problems. Ethical considerations and statistical evaluations and comparisons were also covered. The reader is referred to the conference agenda, speakers, and participants at the end of this appendix for more details.

Speakers' Presentations

As part of the committee's information-gathering process, the conference speakers were asked to discuss recent developments, problems, and research needs in conducting clinical trials with small numbers of participants. In preparing their presentations, the speakers were asked to use two scenarios formulated by the committee during its first committee meeting, namely, (1) clinical trials to prevent bone loss in microgravity and (2) clinical trials on split liver transplantations in patients with human immunodeficiency virus infection and patients with fulminating liver failure. The conference format was organized to achieve balanced times for each speaker's presentation followed by a discussion of the committee with the speakers and invited participants. Overall, the speakers' presentations helped the committee frame the issues and questions in its task of reviewing the methodologies for clinical trials with small sample sizes, determining research gaps and needs, and making recommendations in the development of this area of medical research.

Speakers' Recommended Literature

In a follow-up letter, the committee asked speakers to submit lists of their recommended readings in their specific fields of expertise. They were each asked for a minimum of 10 published articles: 5 of which they are neither an author nor a coauthor and 5 of which they are an author or a coauthor. The speakers' recommended readings are also included in Appendix C and, where relevant, in the References section.

Committee Website and Live Audiocast of Conference

The committee website (http://www.iom.edu/smalln) included a page describing the September 28, 2000, conference. The page served the purpose of disseminating information about the conference to a broader public audience, beyond those professionals who were invited, who might have a stake in the study. The page also allowed comments, suggestions, and questions on the study in general and on the conference in particular to be electronically mailed to Institute of Medicine staff.

The conference was carried on a live audiocast for the benefit of those who were unable to attend. Two weeks before the conference date, a postcard announcement of the live audiocast together with the conference agenda and a one-page description of the conference were sent to invited individuals who had not registered to attend and a wider national audience unlikely to attend. This was done to ensure maximum dissemination of the conference proceedings. After the conference the speakers' visual and audio presentations were posted on the committee's website to allow the widest continuing public access in this phase of the committee's information-gathering activities before the subsequent release of its report to the public.

PREPARING THE REPORT

Discussion of Committee's Charge

At the first of three meetings, the committee reviewed the statement of task, which it accepted with minor changes to make it accurate with regard to statistical terminology and usage. The committee agreed that its composition was sufficient to accomplish the task given the work plan and time schedule of 6 months. In fulfilling the committee's charge, it was anticipated that the study report would serve as a state-of-the science guide to those interested in planning, designing, conducting, and analyzing clinical trials with small numbers participants. The audience for the report was defined to include federal agencies at the policy and program levels, researchers concerned with conducting clinical trials, clinicians, students, patients, and patient advocacy groups.

Discussion of Committee's Charge with Sponsor

In a telephone conference call during its first meeting, the committee discussed with the study sponsor the statement of task. The sponsor presented a summary of the issues that it wanted the committee to address: (1) a critique of the sponsor's proposed methodology on countermeasure evaluation; (2) suggestions for improvements to the proposed methodology or the use of an alternate methodology; and (3) methods for the evaluation of treatments, incorporation of data from surrogate studies, incorporation of treatment compliance information, and sequential decision making on treatment efficacy. The committee determined that, through the invitational conference and its final report, it would be able to meet the sponsor's charge to the committee.

Organization of the Report and Committee Working Groups

The committee agreed to organize the report around four chapters, which included an introduction (Chapter 1), a chapter on design of small clinical trials (Chapter 2), a chapter on statistical approaches to analysis of small clinical trials (Chapter 3), and a concluding chapter on general guidelines on small clinical trials (Chapter 4). Appendices include this one, on study methods, a glossary of statistical and clinical trials terms (Appendix B), a selected bibliography on small clinical trials research (Appendix C), and committee and staff biographies (Appendix D). To facilitate writing of the report, the committee formed two working groups: the clinical trials group and the biostatistical group. The clinical trials group is primarily responsible for the content of Chapter 2, which focused on the design of clinical trials with various numbers of small sample sizes. The biostatistical group is primarily responsible for Chapter 3, which focused on the statistical analyses applied to clinical trials with small sample sizes. The introduction and Appendixes were written or assembled by study staff; the Statistical Analyses section in this appendix was written by the committee, however.

During the third meeting, the committee focused on refining the content of the report and the committee's principal findings and recommendations. Due to the sponsor's imposed time limitation on the study, the committee had only the third meeting to discuss as a group the implications of the information collected. The committee felt that, given the time constraint, it was unable to engage in the amount of deliberation it wished it could to fully meet the task given to the committee for this important and developing area of research. The committee as a whole is responsible for the information included in the entire report.

CONFERENCE AGENDA

"Future Directions for Small n Clinical Research Trials"

National Academy of Sciences Lecture Room
2101 Constitution Avenue, N. W.
Washington, D. C.
September 28, 2000

8:25 a.m. **Opening Remarks**
Suzanne T. Ildstad, Chair of the Committee

8:30 **Overview of the Science of Small *n* Clinical Research Trials**
Martin Delaney, Founding Director, Project Inform

Design and Evaluation of Small *n* Clinical Research Trials

9:00 **Design of Small *n* Clinical Research Trials**
Curtis L. Meinert, Johns Hopkins University School of Public Health

9:30 **Quantitative Assessment of Countermeasure Efficacy for Long-Term Space Missions**
Alan H. Feiveson, Johnson Space Center, NASA

10:00 **Sequential Design**
Nancy Flournoy, The American University

10:30 **Welcome**
Kenneth I. Shine, M.D., President, Institute of Medicine

10:40 **Break**

11:00 **Clinical Trials with *n* of > 1**
Jean Emond, Center for Liver Disease and Transplantation, New York Presbyterian Hospital

11:30 **Small Clinical Research Trials: Needs Beyond Space**
Denise L. Faustman, Massachusetts General Hospital

12:00 **Lunch Break**

Statistical Methodologies for Small *n* Clinical Trials

1:00 p.m. **Meta-Analysis and Alternative Methods**
Betsy J. Becker, Michigan State University

1:30 **Decision Analysis and Small Clinical Trials**
Stephen G. Pauker, New England Medical Center

2:00 **Bayesian Strategies for Small *n* Clinical Trials**
Peter F. Thall, M. D. Anderson Cancer Center, Houston

2:30 ***n* - of - 1 Clinical Trials**
Deborah R. Zucker, New England Medical Center

3:00 **Break**

Development and Monitoring of Small *n* Clinical Trials

3:15 **Research Needs in Developing Small *n* Clinical Trials**
Helena Mishoe, National Heart, Lung and Blood Institute, National Institute of Health

3:45 **Regulatory Issues with Small *n* Clinical Research Trials**
Jay Siegel, Office of Therapeutics Research and Review, Food and Drug Administration

4:15 **Ethical and Patient Information Concerns: Who Goes First?**
Lawrence K. Altman, New York University Medical School and New York Times medical correspondent and author of *Who Goes First?: The Story of Self-Experimentation in Medicine*

4:45 **Closing Remarks**

5:00 **Reception in the Great Hall of the National Academy of Sciences**

ADDITIONAL PARTICIPANTS

Gregory Campbell
Food and Drug Administration
Rockville, MD

Nitza Cintron
Wyle Laboratories
Houston, TX

Janis Davis-Street
NASA
Houston, TX

Lawrence Freedman
National Heart, Lung, and Blood Institute
Bethesda, MD

Carolin Frey
Children's National Medical Center
Washington, DC

Nancy Geller
National Heart, Lung, and Blood Institute
Bethesda, MD

Judith Hayes
Wyle Laboratories
Houston, TX

Eric Leifer
National Heart, Lung, and Blood Institute
Bethesda, MD

Linda Loerch
Wyle Laboratories
Houston, TX

Seigo Ohi
Howard University
Washington, DC

Kantilal Patel
Children's National Medical Center
Washington, DC

Clarence Sams
Wyle Laboratories
Houston, TX

David Samson
Blue Cross Blue Shield Association
Washington, DC

Victor S. Schneider
NASA Headquarters
Washington, DC

Steve Singer
Johns Hopkins University School of Public Health
Baltimore, MD

Mario Stylianou
National Heart, Lung, and Blood Institute
Bethesda, MD

Marlies Van Hoef
Transplant Creations, L. C.
Falls Church, VA

Lakshmi Vishnuvajjala
Food and Drug Administration
Rockville, MD

Teng Weng
Food and Drug Administration
Rockville, MD

Gang Zheng
National Heart, Lung, and Blood Institute
Bethesda, MD

STATISTICAL ANALYSES

Statistical Methods of Drawing Inferences

In the so-called frequentist mode of inference, there are three probabilities of interest, the *p* value, the Type I error probability, and the Type II error probability. In significance testing, as described by R. A. Fisher, the *p* value is the probability of finding results that are at least as far away from the null hypothesis as those actually observed in a given experiment, with respect to the null probability model for the experiment. Note that because the null hypothesis is assumed for the probability model, a *p* value can speak only to how probable or improbable the data are in their departure from expectation under the null hypothesis. The *p* value does not speak to how probable or improbable the null hypothesis is, because to do so immediately takes one outside the probability model generating the data under the null hypothesis (a Bayesian posterior probability addresses this –[see below]). Thus, it is entirely possible that a result can have a small *p* value, indicating that the data are unlikely to be so extreme in their departure from expectation under the null hypothesis, and yet the null hypothesis may itself be very likely. Anyone who has ever gotten a positive result on a screening examination and found that result to be a false positive understands this point: under the null hypothesis of no disease, the probability of a positive screening test result is very small (the *p* value is small and highly significant). With rare diseases, however, most of the positive results are false positives (i.e., the null hypothesis is actually true in most of these cases).

In the Neyman-Pearson paradigm of hypothesis testing, it is imagined that any experiment can be repeated indefinitely, and in each hypothetical replication the null hypothesis will be rejected according to a fixed decision rule. The Type I error describes the long-run proportion of times that the null hypothesis will be so rejected, assuming in each case that it is actually true. The Neyman-Pearson approach also considers various explicit alternative hypotheses and for each one quantifies the Type II error probability, which is the long-run proportion of times that the decision rule will fail to reject the null hypothesis when the given alternative is true.

The interpretation and use of Type I and Type II error probabilities are quite distinct because they are calculated under different hypotheses. The Type I error probability describes the largest *p* value that will be declared statistically significant by chance alone when the null hypothesis is true. Because the Type I error probability gives the long-run proportion of instances in which the decision procedure will err by rejecting a true null hypothesis, it is used to control the occurrence of false positives. The Type II error probability is related to the ability of the test to arrive at a proper rejection of the null hypothesis under any one of the non-null-hypothesis alternatives of interest. The statistical power of a hypothesis test is the probability complementary to the Type II error probability, evaluated at a given alternative, and generally depends on the decision criterion for rejection of the null hypothesis, the probability model for the alternative hypothesis, and the sample size.

The Type II error probability (or, equivalently, the statistical power) is important in the planning stage of an experiment, because it indicates the likelihood that a real phenomenon of interest will be declared statistically significant, thus helping the investigator avoid the time and expense of conducting an experiment that would be hopeless at uncovering the truth. The meaning of a failure to reject the null hypothesis by a low-power test procedure is difficult to interpret, because one cannot distinguish between no true effect or an experimental inability to find one even if it exists. (After an experiment is concluded, however, the Type II error probability has less relevance as a measure of the uncertainty than does a confidence interval or region for the parameter or parameters of interest.)

An important theoretical criticism of all of the above frequentist approaches is that the main questions of scientific inference are not addressed: given the results of an experiment, (i) what is the weight of the evidence in favor of one hypothesis and against another? (ii) what should the investigator believe is true? and (iii) what steps should now be taken? These three questions require different answers.

It is a common misconception that the *p* value is a valid measure of evidence against the null hypothesis—the (misguided) notion being that the smaller the *p* value, the stronger the evidence. Although in many common situations there is a useful correspondence between the *p* value and a proper notion of evidence, there are many other examples in which the *p* value utterly fails to serve as a cogent measure of weight of evidence. There is a strong argument that any measure of evidence must be a relative one (one hypothesis versus another). One sees immediately that the *p* value cannot be a proper measure of the weight of evidence against a null hypothesis relative to a given alternative, because the *p* value entirely ignores all alternatives, being solely concerned with null hypothesis probabilities. Thus, it is entirely possible for an observed *p* value of 0.0001 to be weak evidence against a given null hypothesis (e. g., if the probability of observing the data is even more unlikely to occur under a given alternative).

Although certain technical details are still under discussion, statisticians generally acknowledge that an appropriate measure of the weight of evidence of one hypothesis relative to that of another is provided by the likelihood ratio, which is the probability of the observed data under the first hypothesis divided by the probability of the observed data under the second one. (The probabilities here are point probabilities, not tail probabilities.) As a descriptive device, a likelihood ratio of 8 or more is sometimes taken as "fairly strong" evidence in favor of the first hypothesis relative to the second one, whereas a likelihood ratio of 32 or more would be taken as "strong" evidence. These adjectives and their boundaries are arbitrary, of course, but correspond to useful benchmarks in inferential settings. See Royall (2000) for further discussion and references to these ideas.

For example, in screening a population for a certain disease, suppose the screening test has a sensitivity of 0.90 and a specificity of 0.95. These are values that can be measured in a laboratory setting (e.g., by testing a large number of known patients with the disease and, in another series, a large number of healthy subjects without the disease). What is the weight of evidence in favor of disease as opposed to no disease given a positive test result? The answer is *not* 5 percent, which would be the *p* value (the probability of a rejection of the null hypothesis of no disease given no disease in truth is the complement of the specificity). The likelihood ratio is an arguably better measure of the weight of evidence provided by a positive test result: since the probability of a positive test result under the hypothesis of true disease is 0.90 while the probability of a positive test under the alternative of no disease is $1 - 0.95 = 0.05$, the likelihood ratio is $0.90/0.05 = 18$ in favor of disease. This is an objective measure of the relative likelihood of the data under the two hypotheses and may be taken as a quantitative measure of weight of evidence, which is "fairly strong" in the adjectival descriptive scheme given above.

Should a patient with a positive test result believe he or she has the disease? This is question (ii) above and takes one directly into the Bayesian framework (see Chapter 3). The Bayesian framework allows one to quantify degrees of subjective belief and to combine the "objective" data with "subjective" prior beliefs to arrive at an a posteriori degree of belief in a hypothesis or theory. In the simplest case, the fundamental result of Bayes's theorem states that the posterior odds in favor of one hypothesis relative to another hypothesis is given by the prior odds multiplied by the likelihood ratio. Thus, the Bayesian paradigm reveals the role of the weight of evidence as measured by the likelihood ratio (or the so-called Bayes factor in more complicated settings) as that which increases or decreases one's prior odds in light of the data to yield one's posterior odds (and thus the a posteriori degree of belief). In the screening example, whether or not the patient should believe he or she has the disease depends on the prior degree of belief. If there are no other signs or symptoms for this patient before the screening test, then the prior probability of disease may logically be taken as the general prevalence of the disease in the screened population, which may be low, say, 0.01 for the sake of discussion. In that case the prior odds (degree of belief) would be 0.01/0.99, or approximately 0.0101, which, when multiplied by the "fairly strong" evidentiary likelihood ratio of 18, yields a posterior odds of only 0.1818 in favor of disease, corresponding to a posterior degree of belief of only 15.4 percent in favor of disease. (Even without appealing to subjective degree of belief, this result indicates that about 85 percent of the positive results will be false-positive results in the general population.) On the other hand, if the patient has other symptoms that may be related to the disease (and might have prompted use of the screening test for diagnostic purposes), then the a priori odds on the disease would be correspondingly higher. If the patient or his physician believes that there is a 10 percent chance of disease before the test results are known, then the prior odds of 0.10/0.90 = 1/9 multiplied by the likelihood ratio of 18 yields posterior odds of 2, or an a posteriori degree of belief of 2/3 in favor of disease. This example also illustrates how two experts in a courtroom proceeding can look at the same body of evidence and arrive at opposite conclusions: a given weight of evidence may be convincing to someone with high prior odds, but unpersuasive to another with low prior odds.

Question (iii), what steps should be taken next?, is the subject of formal decision theory discussed in Chapter 3.

The committee concludes this section on statistical methods of drawing inferences with the statement that should be obvious by this point: there is no unique solution to the problem of scientific induction. Consequently, the various ways of drawing statistical inferences and the various probability measures should always be used with some caution, and with a view toward using the methods that are best suited to address the applied problem at hand.

Statistical Derivation of Prediction Limits

The following sections describe statistical derivation of nonparametric, normal, lognormal, and Poisson prediction limits and intervals in some detail, using the astronaut problem as an illustration.

Nonparametric Prediction Limits

Recall that α is the false positive rate for a single endpoint and that α^* is the experiment-wise false positive rate for all k endpoints. Under the conservative assumption of independence, the Bonferroni inequality gives $\alpha = \alpha^*/k$. For simplicity of notation, we do not index the p sets of measurements for each of the k endpoints, only for a single endpoint. Note that in practice, the endpoints may be correlated and the actual confidence level provided by the method will be somewhat higher than the estimated value.

To understand the implications of various design alternatives on the resulting experiment-wise confidence levels, let $y(s_i; n_i)$ denote the s_ith largest value (i.e., order statistic) from the n_i astronauts on spaceflight i ($i = 1, \ldots, p$) and let $x_{(u,n)}$ denote the uth order statistic from a group of control astronauts of size n. One can now express the previous discussion mathematically as

$$\Pr\left\{y_{(s_1,n_1)} > x_{(u,n)}, y_{(s_2,n_2)} > x_{(u,n)}, \ldots, y_{(s_p,n_p)} > x_{(u,n)}\right\} \le \alpha^*,$$

where α^* is the experiment-wise rate of false-positive results (e.g., $\alpha^* = 0.05$). To evaluate the joint probability note that the probability density function of the uth order statistic from a sample of size n [i.e., $x_{(u,n)}$] is

$$g(x,n,u) = \frac{n!}{(u-1)!(n-1)!}\left[F(x)\right]^{u-1}\left[1-F(x)\right]^{n-u} \cdot f(x),$$

where

$$\int_{-\infty}^{\infty}[F(x)]^{u-1}[1-F(x)]^{n-u} \cdot f(x)d(x) = \left[\frac{n!}{(u-1)!(n-u)!}\right]^{-1}$$

$$= \left[\frac{n(n-1)!}{(u-1)!(n-u)!}\right]^{-1}$$

$$= \left[n\binom{n-1}{u-1}\right]^{-1},$$

(Sarhan and Greenberg, 1962). Since

$$\Pr\left\{y_{(j,m)} \ge x\right\} = \sum_{i=0}^{j-1}\binom{m}{i}[F(x)]^{i}[1-F(x)]^{m-i},$$

the joint probability is then

$$\frac{n}{\sum_{i=1}^{p} n_i + n} \sum_{j_1=0}^{s_i-1} \sum_{j_2=0}^{s_2-1} \cdots \sum_{j_p=0}^{s_p-1} \frac{\binom{n_1}{J_1}\binom{n_2}{j_2}\cdots\binom{n_p}{s_p}\binom{n-1}{u-1}}{\binom{\sum_{i=1}^{p} n_i + n - 1}{\sum_{i=1}^{p} j_i + u - 1}} = \alpha,$$

(Chou and Owen, 1986; Gibbons, 1990, 1991, 1994). A lower bound on the probability of the s_ith largest experimental measurement (e.g., the median) in all p spaceflights exceeding the uth largest control measurement for any of the k outcome measures is given by $\alpha^* = 1 - (1 - \alpha)^k$. One minus this probability provides the corresponding confidence level. Ultimately, for practical applications one would typically like the overall confidence level to be approximately 95% (i.e., $\alpha^* \leq 0.05$).

To determine if an outcome measure is significantly decreased in experimental astronauts relative to control astronauts, let $x_{(l,n)}$ denote the lth smallest measurement from the group of control astronauts of size n. Then the equation becomes

$$\Pr\left\lfloor y_{(s_1,n_1)} < x_{(l,n)}, y_{(s_2,n_2)} < x_{(l,n)}, \ldots, y_{(s_p n_p)} < x_{(l,n)} \right\rfloor \leq \alpha^*,$$

which leads to

$$\frac{n}{\sum_{i}^{p} n_i + n} \sum_{j_1=s_1}^{n_i} \sum_{j_2=s_2}^{n_2} \cdots \sum_{j_p=s_p}^{n_p} \frac{\binom{n_1}{J_1}\binom{n_2}{j_2}\cdots\binom{n_p}{j_p}\binom{n-1}{l-1}}{\binom{\sum_{i=1}^{p} n_i + n - 1}{\sum_{i=1}^{p} j_i + l - 1}} = \alpha.$$

The probability of the s_ith largest experimental measurement (e.g., the median) in all p spaceflights being simultaneously less than the lth smallest control measurement for any of the k outcome measures is given by $\alpha^* = 1 - (1 - \alpha)^k$, and 1 minus this probability provides the corresponding confidence level. For a two-sided interval, one can compute upper and lower limits each with probability $\alpha^* /2$. If s_i is the median of the n_i experimental measurements in spaceflight i, then the upper prediction limit can be computed with probability approximately $\alpha^*/2$, and the lower limit is simply the value of the $l = (n - u + 1)$th ordered measurement.

Parametric Prediction Limits

Although nonparametric prediction limits are most general, in certain cases the distributional form of a particular endpoint is well known and a parametric approach is well justified. Most relevant to this type of application are normal, lognormal, and Poisson prediction intervals. The reader is referred to the books by Guttman (1970), Hahn and Meeker (1991), and Gibbons (1994) for a general overview.

Normal Distribution

For the case of a normally distributed endpoint, one can derive an approximate prediction limit by noting that the experiment-wise rate of false positive results α^* can be achieved by setting the individual endpoint rate of false-positive results α equal to

$$\alpha = \left[1-\left(1-\alpha^*\right)^{1/k}\right]^{1/p}.$$

As an example, let α^* equal 0.05 and k equal 10 endpoints. For p equal to 1 (i.e., a single space mission),

$$\alpha = \left[1-\left(1-.05\right)^{1/10}\right]^{1/1} = 0.005,$$

which would lead to quite limited statistical power to detect a significant difference for any single endpoint. By contrast, with p equal 2 (i.e., two space missions),

$$\alpha = \left[1-\left(1-.05\right)^{1/10}\right]^{1/2} = 0.072,$$

which would require a much smaller effect size to declare a significant difference. With p equal to 3

$$\alpha = \left[1-\left(1-.05\right)^{1/10}\right]^{1/3} = 0.172,$$

which can be used to detect an even smaller difference. Assuming normality, the 100 (1 – α) percent upper prediction limit (UPL) for the mean of the n_i experimental subjects in replicate i, for $i = 1, \ldots, p$, is given by

$$\text{UPL} = \bar{x} + t_{(n-1,1-\alpha)}s\sqrt{\frac{1}{n_i}+\frac{1}{n}},$$

where $\bar{x}$ and s are the means and standard deviation of the n control measurements, respectively, and t is the $1-\alpha$ upper percentage point of Student's t – distribution on $n-1$ degrees of freedom. For example, if n is equal to 20, n_i is equal to 5, p is equal to 3, and k is equal to 10, then the prediction limit is

$$\text{UPL} = \bar{x} + 0.97s\sqrt{\frac{1}{5}+\frac{1}{20}} = \bar{x} + 0.49s.$$

By contrast, with p = 1, the corresponding prediction limit is almost three times larger, i.e.,

$$\text{UPL} = \bar{x} + 2.86s\sqrt{\frac{1}{5}+\frac{1}{20}} = \bar{x} + 1.43s.$$

The corresponding lower prediction limit (LPL) is given by

$$\text{LPL} = \bar{x} - t_{(n-1,1-\alpha)}s\sqrt{\frac{1}{n_i}+\frac{1}{n}},$$

and the two-sided prediction interval (PI) is

$$\text{PI} = \bar{x} \pm t_{(n-1,1-\alpha/2)}s\sqrt{\frac{1}{n_i}+\frac{1}{n}}.$$

Note that this solution is approximate because it ignores the dependency introduced by comparing each of the p source sets with the same control group. The magnitude of the correlation is

$$r_{ij} = 1\Big/\sqrt{\left(\frac{n}{n_i}+1\right)\left(\frac{n}{n_j}+1\right)}.$$

For n equal to 20 and n_i equal to n_j which is equal to 5, the correlation (r) is 0.2. Incorporation of this correlation into the computation of the prediction limit is complex and requires computation of the relevant critical values from a multivariate t - distribution (Dunnett, 1955; Gibbons, 1994). The approximate prediction limits presented above, which assume independence, will slightly overestimate the true values that incorporate the dependence, but are much easier to compute.

Lognormal Prediction Limits

Note that it is often tempting to attempt to bring about normality by transforming the raw data and then applying the above method to the transformed data. A natural choice is to take natural logarithms of the raw data, compute the normal limit on the transformed data, and exponentiate the resulting limit estimate. Although this is a perfectly reasonable approach, it should be noted that the exponentiated limit is for the geometric mean of the n_i experimental sources (i.e., the median) and not the arithmetic mean intensity, which will always be larger than the median if the data are, in fact, from a lognormal distribution. Nevertheless, this can be a useful strategy if the raw intensity data are highly skewed. Bhaumik and Gibbons (submitted for publication) have developed a lognormal prediction limit for the mean of n_i future samples.

Poisson Distribution

For endpoints that are the result of a counting process, a Poisson distribution may be a reasonable choice for statistical purposes. To construct such a limit estimate, assume that y, the sum of n control measurements, has a Poisson distribution with mean μ. Having observed y one needs to predict y^*, the sum of n_i experimental measurements, which has a Poisson distribution with mean $c\mu$ In the present context, c is equal to n_i/n. On the basis of a result of Cox and Hinkley (1974), Gibbons (1987) derived the corresponding UPL for y^* as

$$\mathrm{UPL}(y^*) = cy + \frac{z^2 c}{2} + zc\sqrt{y\left(1+\frac{1}{c}\right)+\frac{z^2}{4}},$$

where z is the $100(1-\alpha)$ percentage point of the normal distribution. In this context, the prediction limit represents an upper bound on the sum of the measurements of the n_i experimental subjects in replicate i and α is defined in the first equation in the section Normal Distribution. The experimental condition is only considered significantly different from control only if the sum of the n_i experimental measurements exceeds the UPL for y^* in all p experimental replicates (e.g., space missions). The corresponding LPL

$$\mathrm{LPL}(y^*) = cy + \frac{z^2 c}{2} - zc\sqrt{y\left(1+\frac{1}{c}\right)+\frac{z^2}{4}},$$

and the two-sided PI is obtained by substituting $z\,[1-\alpha/2]$ into the previous two equations.

The General Linear Hierarchical Regression Model

To describe the general linear hierarchical regression model in a general way for data that are either clustered or longitudinal, the terminology of multilevel analysis can be used (Goldstein, 1995). For this, let i denote the Level - 2 units (clusters in the clustered data context or subjects in the longitudinal data context), and let j denote the Level - 1 units (subjects in the clustered data context or repeated observations in the longitudinal data context). Assume that there are $i = 1, \ldots N$ Level - 2 units and $j = 1, \ldots; n_i$ Level - 1 units nested within each Level - 2 unit. The mixed-effects regression model for the n_i x 1 response vector **y** for Level - 2 unit i (subject or cluster) can be written as

$$\mathbf{y_i} = \mathbf{W_i}\alpha + \mathbf{X_i}\beta_i + \varepsilon_i \qquad i = 1,\ldots N,$$

where $\mathbf{W_i}$ is a known n_i x p design matrix for the fixed effects, α is the p x 1 vector of unknown fixed regression parameters, $\mathbf{X_i}$ is a known n_i x r design matrix for the random effects, and β_i is the r x 1 vector of random individual effects, and ε_i is the n_i x 1 error vector. The distribution of the random effects is typically assumed to be multivariate normal with mean vector 0 and covariance matrix Σ, and the errors are assumed to be independently distributed as multivariate normal with mean vector 0 and covariance matrix $\Sigma\varepsilon = \sigma_\varepsilon^2 \Omega_i$. Although Ω_i carries the subscript i, it depends on i only through its dimension n_i, that is, the number of parameters in Ω_i will not depend on i. In the case of independent residuals, Ω_i is equal to I_i, but for the case of longitudinal designs, one can define ω to be the s x 1 vector of autocorrelation matrix (Chi and Reinsel, 1989).

Different types of correlation structures have been considered including the first-order autoregressive process AR(1), the first-order moving average process MA(1), the first-order mixed autoregressive-moving average process ARMA(1,1), and the general autocorrelation structure. A typical assumption in models with correlation structures is that the variance of the errors is constant over time and that the covariance of errors from different time points depends only on the time interval between these time points and not on the starting time point. This assumption, referred to as the *stationarity assumption*, is assumed for the aforementioned forms. Another form of correlation structures is described by Mansour and colleagues (1985), who examine correlation structures that follow the first-order autoregressive process, however, where the assumption of *stationarity* is relaxed.

As a result of the above assumptions, the observations $\mathbf{y_i}$ and random coefficients β have the joint multivariate normal distribution

$$\begin{bmatrix} y_i \\ \beta_i \end{bmatrix} \sim N\left(\begin{bmatrix} W_i\alpha \\ 0 \end{bmatrix}, \begin{bmatrix} X_i\Sigma_\beta X_i' + \sigma^2{}_\varepsilon\Omega_i & X_i\Sigma_\beta \\ \Sigma_\beta X_i' & \Sigma_\beta \end{bmatrix} \right).$$

The mean of the posterior distribution of β, given $\mathbf{y}_i$, yields the empirical Bayes (EB) or EAP (expected a posteriori) estimator of the Level 2 random parameters,

$$\bar{\beta}_i = \left[\mathbf{X}_i' \left(\sigma_\varepsilon^2 \Omega_i \right)^{-1} \mathbf{X}_i + \Sigma_\beta^{-1} \right]^{-1} \mathbf{X}_i' \left(\sigma_\varepsilon^2 \Omega_i \right)^{-1} \left(y_i - W_i \alpha \right),$$

with the corresponding posterior covariance matrix given by

$$\Sigma_{\beta | y_i} = \left[X_i' \left(\sigma_\varepsilon^2 \Omega_i \right)^{-1} X_i + \Sigma_\beta^{-1} \right]^{-1}.$$

Details regarding estimation of $\sum_\beta$, α, σ^2_ε and ω were originally introduced by Laird and Ware (1982).

Empirical Bayes Methods and Risk-Based Allocation

Why are empirical Bayes methods needed for analysis of experiments with risk-based allocation? There are two reasons: first, the natural heterogeneity from subject to subject requires some accounting for random effects; and second, the differential selection of groups due to the risk-based allocation is handled perfectly by the "u - v" method introduced by Herbert Robbins. This section considers both of these ideas in a little detail.

Consider the following simple model. Let a be a prespecified nonnegative integer, and let X be a count variable observed pretreatment. Given an unobservable nonnegative random variable θ, which varies in an arbitrary and unknown manner in the population of subjects under study, assume that X has a Poisson distribution with mean θ. Now, let Y be another count variable, observed postreatment, and given both X and θ, we suppose that Y has a Poisson distribution with mean $c_0\theta$ if X *is* $\leq a$ or mean $c_1\theta$ if X is $>a$. In symbols, $X|\theta \sim \mathbf{P}(\theta)$, $\theta \sim G(\theta)$ unknown, and $Y|X, \theta \sim \mathbf{P}(c_{I(X)}\theta)$, where the index $I(X) = I[X > a]$ is the indicator that X exceeds a. This model reflects the risk-based allocation design: if X is $\leq a$ the subject is at low risk and the standard treatment is given, where the treatment is assumed to operate multiplicatively on θ by the effect size c_0, whereas if X is $>a$, the subject is at high risk and an experimental treatment is given, where the treatment is again assumed to operate on θ multiplicatively, but with a possibly different effect size, c_1. (In the risk-based design, one does not need to assume the Poisson distribution for Y given X and θ, but only that the conditional mean of Y satisfies $E[Y|X, \theta] = c_{I(X)}\theta$. The Poisson assumption is made for convenience in this discussion.) How can one estimate the effect sizes c_0 and c_1 in light of the fact that θ is an unobservable trait of the subjects with unknown distribution?

Notice that θ usually cannot be ignored and a simple model for Y as a function of X is assumed. This is because the correct mean of Y given X alone is seen upon integration to be $E[Y|X] = c_{I(X)}E[\theta|X]$, but the mean of θ for given values of X can be a highly complicated function and is generally unknown since the distribution G is unknown. The only distributions on θ for which $E[\theta|X]$ is a simple linear function of X is the family of gamma distributions, the so-called conjugate prior for the Poisson distribution. Unless there is an empirical basis for assuming the conjugate prior, however, the posterior mean of θ given X will not be linear. (This simple fact is what separates empirical Bayes methods from subjective Bayes methods, in which a gamma prior would often be assumed, gratuitously in many cases.)

A simple ratio of averages also cannot be taken because of the different treatments. If there were only a single treatment (the case in which a is equal to ∞), one could estimate c_0 consistently by the ratio of the average Y to the average X, because $E[Y] = E\{E[Y|X, \theta]\} = E\{c_0\theta\} = c_0E[\theta] = c_0E[X]$. Where there are two treatment effects for $X \leq a$ and $X > a$, however, it can be shown that $avg\{Y\}/avg\{X\}$ is an inconsistent (biased) estimator of both treatment effects. A better tool is needed.

Enter the Robbins *u-v* method. Robbins and Zhang (1991) proved the following theorem. If $u(x)$ is any known function, then under the assumption $X|\theta \sim P(\theta)$, with the distribution of θ arbitrary, the expected value of θ times $u(X)$ is $E[\theta u(X)] = E[Xu(X\text{-}1)]$. This result is called the fundamental empirical Bayes identity for the Poisson case and is remarkable because it expresses an unknown expectation of an unobservable quantity on the left in terms of an expectation of an entirely observable, hence estimable, quantity on the right.[1] Here's how this result is applied to the problem. First, let $u(x) = I[x \leq a]$ be the indicator that standard treatment has been assigned. One finds an expression for treatment effect c_0 as follows. First, note that $E[Y\theta(X)|X, q] = u(X)c_0\theta$, because the expression is non-zero only for $X \leq a$. Taking expectations of both sides with respect to the joint distribution of X and θ, and applying the fundamental identity, one finds

$$E[Yu(X)] = c_0E[\theta u(X)] = c_0E[Xu(X - 1)] = c_0E\{XI[X \leq a+1]\}.$$

Consequently, one has $c_0 = E\{YI[X \leq a]\}/E\{XI[X \leq a + 1]\}$, which can easily be estimated: simply sum the values of the endpoint Y among those subjects with $X \leq a$ and divide by the sum of the values of X among all those

[1] The *u-v* method of estimation gets its name because Robbins considered problems in which for a given function $u(x)$ there is another function $\nu(x)$ such that $E[\theta u(X)]$ is equal to $E[\nu(X)]$. In the Poisson case, the equation is $\nu(x) = xu(x\text{-}1)$.

with $X \leq a + 1$ at the baseline. The Law of Large Numbers ensures that the ratio is a consistent estimator as the sample size of subjects increases.

As an illustration, consider the motorist example presented in Box 2-6 in Chapter 2. Suppose one wanted to find out if there was a multiplicative temporal effect on the accident-proneness parameter θ between year 1 and year 2 for the subset of drivers with zero accidents. This is the case in which a is equal to 0. The empirical Bayes estimate of c_0 is given by the observed total number of accidents in year 2 (γ) for those with zero accidents in year 1 ($X = 0$), divided by the sum of the values of X among all those with $X \leq 1$ in year 1, which is just the number of drivers with exactly one accident at the baseline. Thus, the prediction procedure discussed in Chapter 2 under the assumption that c_0 is equal to 1 has been converted into an estimation procedure for treatment effect in an assured allocation design. If an active treatment rather than simply the passage of time was applied, its effect would be included in the parameter c_0.

An analogous result applies for estimation of c_1 among the high-risk subjects with $a > 1$. In this case $c_1 = E\{YI[X > a]\}/E\{XI[X > a{+}1]\}$, which can be estimated by summing the values of the endpoint Y among those subjects with $X > a$, and dividing by the sum of the values of X among all those with $X > a + 1$ at the baseline. For example, the temporal effect on accident proneness for those drivers with one or more accidents in the baseline year can be estimated by the observed total number of accidents in the next year among those with one or more accidents in the baseline year divided by the total number of accidents suffered by all those with two or more accidents in the year baseline (and the denominator is an unbiased predictor of the numerator under the null hypothesis c_1 is equal to *1*).

The above theory is called *semiparametric* because of the parametric Poisson assumption and the nonparametric assumption concerning the distribution of θ. The committee closes this section with some remarks on a completely *nonparametric* estimation procedure with use of an auxiliary variable. The assumption that X has a Poisson distribution is now dropped, with only the assumption retained that whatever the distribution of X given θ, $E[X|\theta]$ is equal to θ. This is really just a definition of θ. For the endpoint variable Y, assume a model for expectations that encompasses both an additive and a multiplicative effect model for standard treatment:

$$E_0[Y \mid X,\theta] = a + bX + c\theta,$$

where the subscript on the expectation indicates standard treatment. The model allows the expectation of Y to depend on X because treatment modality (e.g., the dosage of a standard therapeutic drug) may depend on the observed baseline measurement. In the risk-based design, one wants to use the model to estimate the mean response for those at higher risk (with, say, $X > a$) under standard treatment, but note that just as in the Poisson case, the model for Y given X alone is generally not a linear model in X, because generally $E[\theta|X]$ is not linear in X, unless θ has a conjugate prior relative to X.

Now assume that there is an auxiliary variable, X', also measured before treatment. X' may be a replicate measurement of X (e.g., a second blood assay), a concomitant measure of risk, or a baseline version of the endpoint Y. X' need not be independent of X, even conditionally given θ. It is assumed that X' is similar to Y in the sense that for some constants a', b', and $c' \neq 0$,

$$E[X' | X, \theta] = a' + b'X + c'\theta,$$

It follows that the variable $Y - (c/c')X'$ does have a simple linear expectation in X:

$$E_0[Y - (c/c')X' | X] = a^* + b^* X,$$

where a^* *is equal to* $a - (c/c')a'$ and b^* is equal to $b - (c/c')b'$. If the ratio c/c' is known, the model can be used with ordinary estimates of a^* and b^* from the subjects on standard treatment to estimate (predict) what the high-risk patients would have yielded for $Y - (c/c')X'$. The treatment effect is estimated using observed values of $Y - (c/c^1)X^1$ together with the relation

Treatment effect $= E_1[Y|X > a] - E_0[Y|X > a] = E_1[Y - (c/c')X'|X > a] - E_0[Y - (c/c')X'|X > a]$

which holds because the expectations of X' given X are the same under E_0 or E_1 as both X and X' are measured pretreatment. If the ratio c/c^1 is not known, it can be estimated for the subjects under standard treatment by special methods (details omitted).

In the cholestyramine example (see Box 2-7), the allocation variable X was a baseline measurement of the total serum cholesterol level. The auxiliary variable X' was another measurement of the total serum cholesterol level taken 4 months after all subjects were given dietary recommendations but before randomization to cholestyramine or placebo. The analysis assumed the ratio c/c' *was equal to 1*, so that the simple change scores $Y - X'$ were linearly related to X, even though Y itself would generally be a nonlinear function of X. Then the treatment effect of cholestyramine versus placebo among the high cholesterol subjects was estimated by the observed average of $Y - X'$ among those taking cholestyramine minus the predicted value of $Y - X'$ among the same patients if they had taken placebo, with the latter quantity estimated by $a^* + b^*X$ evaluated at the average values of X among the subjects with high cholesterol levels. For further details, see Finkelstein et al. (1996) and Robbins (1993).

These results often surprise even the best statisticians. Robbins' general empirical Bayes theory is both elegant and nontrivial. In the Poisson case the point and interval predictions of the number of accidents to be had in year 2 by those drivers with zero accidents in year 1 are applications of general (i.e., semiparametric) empirical Bayes theorems for mixtures of Poisson random variables. The interested reader may want to consider the results in a little more detail. Let the random variable X denote the number of accidents in year 1 for a given motorist and let random variable Y denote the number of accidents in year 2 for the same motorist. Let random variable q denote the unobservable accident proneness parameter for that motorist. The model under consideration makes three assumptions:

(i) θ has an unknown distribution G with finite expectation;
(ii) given θ, the distribution of X is Poisson with mean θ; and
(iii) given X and θ, the distribution of Y is also Poisson with mean θ.

Assumption (iii) is the null assumption that road conditions and driving habits remain constant. The assumption implies that θ alone determines the distribution of Y, irrespective of X. X and Y are unconditionally correlated in ignorance of θ.

Now, let $u(x)$ be any function of x. Two fundamental empirical Bayes identities for Poisson random variables due to Robbins can be stated:

First-order empirical Bayes identity for Poisson variables:

$$E[u(X)\theta] = E[Xu(X-1)],$$

where the expectation is taken with respect to the joint distribution of X and θ determined by (i) and (ii).

Second-order empirical Bayes identity for Poisson variables:

$$E[u(X)\theta^2] = E[X(X-1)u(X-2)].$$

The proofs of these assertions are elementary: one demonstrates them first for conditional expectations given θ, pointwise for each θ. Then one takes expectations with respect to G (details omitted).

In the application, let $u(x)$ equal I[x equal 0], the indicator function for x equal to 0. The key result for the point prediction is

$$E\{YI[X=0]\} = P[X=1].$$

To see this, write $E[Yu(X)|X, \theta] = u(X)E[Y|X, \theta] = u(X)\theta$. Take expectations with respect to (X, θ) and use the first identity: $E[Yu(X)] = E[u(X)\theta] = E[Xu(X-1)] = E\{XI[X=1]\} = P[X=1]$.

Thus in a population of n drivers, the predicted number of accidents in year 2 among zero-accident drivers in year 1 is

$$E\{\Sigma_i Y_i I[X_i = 0]\} = nP[X=1],$$

and using the sample estimate of $P[X = 1]$, namely (number of drivers with one accident)/n, one can conclude that the prediction is the number of drivers with exactly one accident in year 1. For the 95 percent prediction interval, the key result is that

$$E\{[Yu(X) - u(X \quad 1)]\}^2 = E\{YI[X=0] - I[X=1]\}^2 = 2\{P[X=1] + P[X=2]\}.$$

The proof is as follows. Conditional on (X, θ),

$$E\{[Yu(X) - u(X-1)]^2 \mid X, 0\} =$$
$$E[Y^2 u(X)^2 \mid X, 0] - 2u(X)u(X-1)E[Y \mid X, \theta] + u(X-1)^2 =$$
$$u(X)^2(\theta + \theta^2) - 2u(X)u(X-1)\theta + u(X-1)^2.$$

The property var$(Y|X, \theta) = E[Y|X, \theta]$ was used for Poisson variables in the first term. By using $u(x)$ equal to $I[x = 0]$, the right-hand side reduces to $I[X=0](\theta + \theta^2) + I[X=1]$. Thus, unconditionally, $E\{[Yu(X) - u(X-1)]^2\} = E\{I[X=0]\theta\} + E\{I[X=0]\theta^2\} + P[X=1]$, and using the first and second fundamental identities, this reduces to

$$E\{XI[X=1]\} + E\{X(X \quad 1)I[X=2]\} + P[X=1] = 2\{P[X=1] + P[X=2]\}.$$

Thus, in a population of n drivers, the mean squared error of prediction is

$$E[\Sigma_i\{Y_i I[X_I = 0] \quad I[X_I = 1]\}^2] = 2n\{P[X=1] + P[X=2]\},$$

which is consistently estimated by twice the number of drivers with exactly one or two accidents in year 1, as used in the 95 percent prediction interval in the report by Finkelstein and Levin (1990).

APPENDIX REFERENCES

Bhaumik, D. K., and R. D. Gibbons. An upper prediction limit for the arithmetic mean of a lognormal random variable. Submitted for publication.

Chi, E. M., and G. C. Reinsel. 1989. Models of longitudinal data with random effects and AR(1) errors. *Journal of the American Statistical Association* 84:452–459.

Chou, Y., and D. Owen. 1986. One-sided distribution-free simultaneous prediction limits for *p* future samples. *Journal of Quality Technology* 18:96–98.

Cox, D. R., and D. V. Hinkley. 1974. *Theoretical Statistics.* London: Chapman & Hall.

Dunnett, C. W. 1955. A multiple comparisons procedure for comparing several treatments with a control. *Journal of the American Statistical Association* 50:1096–1121.

Finkelstein, M. O., andd B. Levin. 1990. *Statistics for Lawyers.* New York: Springer Verlag.

Finkelstein, M. O., B. Levin, and H. Robbins. 1996. Clinical and prophylactic trials with assured new treatment for those at greater risk. Part II. Examples. *American Journal of Public Health* 86:696–705.

Gibbons, R. D. 1987. Statistical models for the analysis of volatile organic compounds in waste disposal sites. *Ground Water* 25:572–580.

Gibbons, R. D. 1990. A general statistical procedure for ground-water detection monitoring at waste disposal facilities. *Ground Water* 28:235–243.

Gibbons, R. D. 1991. Some additional nonparametric prediction limits for ground-water detection monitoring at waste disposal facilities. *Ground Water* 29:729–736.

Gibbons, R. D. 1994. *Statistical Methods for Groundwater Monitoring.* New York: Wiley.

Goldstein, H. 1995. *Multilevel Statistical Models*, 2nd ed. New York: Halstead Press.

Guttman, I. 1970. *Statistical Tolerance Regions: Classical and Bayesian.* Darien, Conn: Hafner.

Hahn, G. J., and W. O. Meeker. 1991. *Statistical Intervals: A Guide for Practitioners.* New York: Wiley.

Laird, N. M., and J. H. Ware. 1982. Random effects models for longitudinal data. *Biometrics* 38:963–974.

Mansour, H., E. V. Nordheim, and J. J. Rutledge. 1985. Maximum likelihood estimation of variance components in repeated measures designs assuming autoregressive errors. *Biometrics* 41:287–294.

Robbins, H. 1993. Comparing two treatments under biased allocation. *La Gazette des Sciences Mathematics du Quebec.* 15:35–41.

Robbins, H., and C. H. Zhang. 1991. Estimating a multiplicative treatment effect under biased allocation. *Biometrika* 78:349–354.

Royall, R. 2000. On the probability of observing misleading statistical evidence. *Journal of the American Statistical Association* 95:760–768 (Discussion, pp. 768–780).

Sarhan, A. and B. Greenberg. 1962. *Contributions to Order Statistics.* New York: Wiley.

Appendix B Glossary of Statistical and Clinical Trials Terms

Acceptance region The set of values of a test statistic for which the null hypothesis is not rejected.

Acceptance sampling A sampling method by which the sample is taken from groups or batches as they pass a specified time point, e.g., age, followed by sampling of individuals within the sampled groups.

Acquired immunodeficiency syndrome (AIDS) The late clinical stage of infection with human immunodeficiency virus (HIV), recognized as a distinct syndrome in 1981.The surveillance definition includes HIV-infected persons who have less than 200 CD4 + T lymphocytes per μL or a CD4 + T lymphocyte percentage of total lymphocytes of less than 14 percent, accompanied by any of 26 clinical conditions (e.g., opportunistic infection, Kaposi's sarcoma, wasting syndrome).

Adaptive cluster sampling A procedure in which an initial set of subjects is selected by a sampling procedure and, whenever the variable of interest of a selected subject satisfies a given criterion, additional subjects whose values are in the neighborhood of those for that subject are added to the sample.

Adaptive sampling A sampling procedure in which the selection process depends on the observed values of some variables of interest.

Additive effect A term used when the effect of administering two treatments together is the sum of their separate effects.

Additive model A model in which the combined effect of several factors is the sum of the effects that would be produced by each of the factors in the absence of the others.

Adjustment A procedure for summarization of a statistical measure in which the effects of differences in composition of the population being compared have been minimized by statistical methods. Examples are adjustment by regression analysis and by standardization. See *standardization.*

Adverse event An undesirable or unwanted consequence experienced by a subject during a clinical trial irrespective of the relationship to the study treatment.

Age standardization A procedure for adjusting rates, e.g., death rates, designed to minimize the effects of differences in age composition when comparing rates for different populations.

Algorithm Any systematic process that consists of an ordered sequence of steps in which each step depends on the outcome of the previous one.

Algorithm, clinical An explicit description of steps to be taken in patient care in specified circumstances.

Alpha (α) The probability of a Type I error. The value of a is usually 0.05. See *significance level.*

Alternative hypothesis The hypothesis against which the null hypothesis is tested.

Analysis of covariance (ANCOVA) An extension of the analysis of variance that allows consideration of the possible effects of covariates on the response variable, in addition to the effects of the factor or treatment variables. The covariates are assumed to be unaffected by treatments, and in general, their relationship to the response is assumed to be linear.

Analysis of variance (ANOVA) A statistical technique that isolates and assesses the contributions of categorical independent variables to variations in the mean value of a continuous dependent variable. The total variance of a set of observations are partitioned according to different factors, e.g., sex, age, treatment groups, and compared by way of *F tests.* Differences between means can then be assessed.

Arc sin transformation A transformation of the form 2 arc sin $\sqrt{p}$, used to stabilize the variance of a binomial random variable.

Area sampling A sampling method in which a geographical region is subdivided into smaller areas (counties, villages, city blocks, etc.), some of which are selected at random, and the chosen areas are then subsampled or completely surveyed. See *cluster sampling.*

Area under curve (AUC) A useful way of summarizing the information from a series of measurements made on an individual over time or for a *dose-response curve*. Calculated by adding the areas under the curve between each pair of consecutive observations, using for example, the *trapezium rule*.

Arithmetic mean The sum of all the values in a set of measurements divided by the number of values in the set.

Assigned treatment The treatment designated to be given to a patient in a clinical trial as indicated at the time of enrollment.

Association Statistical dependence between two or more events, characteristics, or other variables. Most often applied in the context of binary variables forming a two-by-two contingency table. A positive association between two variables exists when the occurrence of higher values of a variable is associated with the occurrence of higher values of another variable. A negative association exists when the occurrence of higher values of one variable is associated with lower values of the other variable.

Assumptions The conditions under which statistical techniques give valid results.

Attack rate The cumulative incidence of a disease or condition in a particular group, during a limited period of time, or under special circumstances such as an epidemic.

Attributable risk A measure of the association between exposure to a particular factor and the risk of a particular outcome, calculated as:

$$\frac{\text{incidence rate among exposed} - \text{incidence rate among unexposed}}{\text{incidence rate among exposed}}$$

Attrition The loss of subjects over the period of a longitudinal study. See *missing values*.

Average An average value represents or summarizes the relevant features of a set of values, and in this sense the term includes the median and the mode.

Balanced design An experimental design in which the same number of observations is taken for each combination of the experimental factors.

Bar chart A graphical representation for displaying discrete data organized in such a way that each observation can fall into one and only one category of the variable. Frequencies are listed along one axis, and categories of the variable are listed along the other axis. The frequencies of each group of observations are represented by the lengths of the corresponding bars. See *histogram*.

Baseline data A set of data collected at the beginning of a study.

Bathtub curve The shape taken by the hazard rate for the event of death in humans. It is relatively high during the first year of life, decreases fairly soon to a minimum, and begins to climb again sometime around ages 45 to 50.

Bayesian confidence interval An interval of a posterior distribution such that the density at any point inside the interval is greater than the density at any point outside. For any probability level, there is generally only one such interval, which is often known as the highest posterior density region.

Bayesian inference Statistical inference based on Bayes's theorem. The focus of the Bayesian approach is the probability distribution of any unknowns, given available information. The process deals with probabilities of hypotheses and probability distributions of parameters, which are not taken into account in classical statistical inference.

Bayes's theorem A theorem in probability theory named after Thomas Bayes (1702–1761), an English clergyman and mathematician. It is a procedure for revising and updating the probability of some event in the light of new evidence. In its simplest form, the theorem is written in terms of conditional probabilities as:

$$P(A|B) = \frac{P(B|A)P(A)}{P(B)}$$

where $P(A|B)$ denotes the conditional probability of event A conditional on event B. The overall probability of an event among a population before knowing the presence or absence of new evidence is called *prior probability*. The updated probability of the event after receiving new information is called *posterior probability*.

Bell-shaped distribution A probability distribution having the overall shape of a vertical cross-section of a bell. Examples are normal distribution and Student's t distribution.

Benefit-cost ratio The ratio of net present value of measurable benefits to costs. Calculation of a benefit-cost ratio is used to determine the economic feasibility or success of a program.

Beta (b) The probability of a Type II error.

Bias Deviation of results or inferences from the truth or processes leading to such a deviation. Any trend in the collection, analysis, interpretation, publication, or review of data that can lead to conclusions that are systematically different from the truth. Statistical bias occurs when the extent to which the statistical method used in a study does not estimate the quantity thought to be estimated or does not test the hypothesis to be tested.

Bimodal distribution A probability distribution or a frequency distribution with two modes.

Binary sequence A sequence whose elements take one of only two possible values, usually denoted 0 or 1.

Binary variable A variable having only two possible values, usually labeled 0 or 1. Data involving this type of variable often require specialized statistical techniques such as logistic regression.

Binomial distribution The probability distribution of the number of occurrences of a binary event in a sample of n independent observations. The distribution is associated with two mutually exclusive outcomes, e.g., death or survival, success or failure.

Bioassay The quantitative evaluation of the potency of a substance by assessing its effects on tissues, cells, live experimental animals, or humans.

Bioequivalence The degree to which clinically important outcomes of treatment by a new preparation resemble those of a previously established preparation.

Bioequivalence trials Trials carried out to compare two or more formulations of a drug containing the same active ingredient to determine whether the different formulations give rise to comparable levels in blood.

Biological efficacy The effect of treatment for all persons who receive the therapeutic agent to which they were assigned. It measures the biological action of a treatment among compliant persons.

Biological plausibility The criterion that an observed, presumably or putatively causal association fits previously existing biological or medical knowledge.

Biometry The application of statistical methods to the study of numerical data on the basis of observations of biological phenomena.

Biostatistics The application of statistical methods to biological and medical problems.

Biplots A graphical display of multivariate data designed to show any structure, pattern, or relationship between variables.

Bit A unit of information consisting of one binary digit.

Bivariate data Data in which the subjects each have measurements on two variables.

Bivariate distribution The joint distribution of two random variables, x and y.

Blinding A procedure used in clinical trials to avoid the possible bias that might be introduced if the patient or doctor, or both, knew which treatment the patient would be receiving. A trial is double blind if both patient and doctor are not aware of treatment given; if either the doctor or the patient is not aware of treatment given, the trial is single blind. Also called *masking*.

Block A term used in experimental design to refer to a homogeneous grouping of experimental units designed to enable the experimenter to isolate and, if necessary, eliminate variability due to extraneous causes.

Block randomization A random allocation procedure used to keep the numbers of subjects in the different groups of a clinical trial closely balanced at all times.

Blot, Western, Northern, Southern Varieties of tests using electrophoresis, nucleic acid base pairing, or protein-antibody interaction to detect and identify DNA or RNA in samples. The Southern blot is used to identify a specific segment of DNA in a sample. The Northern blot detects and identifies samples of RNA. The Western blot is widely used in a test for detection of human immunodeficiency virus infection.

Bootstrap A data-based simulation method for statistical inference that can be used to study the variability of estimated characteristics of the probability distribution of a set of observations and provide confidence intervals for parameters in situations in which these are difficult or impossible to derive in the usual way.

Bonferroni correction A procedure for guarding against an increase in the Type I error when performing multiple significance tests. To maintain the Type I error at some selected value, a, each of the m tests to be performed is judged against a significance level, a/m. This method is acceptable for a small number of simultaneous tests to be performed (up to five).

Causality The relating of causes to the effects that they produce. A cause is termed "necessary" when it must always precede an effect. This effect need not be the sole result of the one cause. A cause is termed "sufficient" when it inevitably initiates or produces an effect. Any given cause may be necessary, sufficient, neither necessary nor sufficient, or both necessary and sufficient.

Censored observation Observation with an unknown value due to the occurrence of an event (e.g., death, loss to follow-up, or termination of study) before the occurrence of the event of interest in the study.

Central limit theorem The tendency for the sampling distribution of means to be a normal (Gaussian) distribution, even if the data do not have a Gaussian distribution, for sufficiently large numbers of subjects.

Central range The range within which the central 90 percent of values of a set of observations lie.

Central tendency A property of the distribution of a variable usually measured by statistics such as the mean, median, and mode.

Chimerism In genetics, the presence in an individual of cells of different origin, such as of blood cells derived from a dizygotic cotwin.

Chi-square distribution The probability distribution of the sum of squares of a number of independent standard normal variables.

Chi-square test Any statistical test based on comparison of a test statistic to a chi-square distribution. The most common chi-square tests (e.g., the Mantel-Haenszel and Pearson chi-square tests) are used to detect whether two or more population distributions differ from one another. These tests usually involve counts of data and may involve comparison of samples from the distribution under study or comparison of a sample to a theoretically expected distribution.

Chi-square test for trend A test applied to a two-dimensional contingency table in which one variable has two categories and the other has *k* ordered categories to assess whether there is a difference in the trend of the proportions in the two groups.

Clinical decision analysis A procedure designed to provide insight into the structure of a clinical problem and to identify the main determinants of diagnostic and therapeutic choice. This procedure is useful to small numbers of clinical cases, even to a single patient (see *n*-of-1 study). The procedure has four stages:

1. Definition of the clinical problem and structuring it as a decision tree. This includes description of the patient, of the possible diagnostic and therapeutic actions, and of the possible outcomes after treatment.
2. Estimation of probabilities for diagnostic and therapeutic outcomes.
3. Performance of the requisite computations for determination of the preferred course of action.
4. Presentation of the results of the analysis in a clinically useful way.

Clinical epidemiology Epidemiological study conducted in a clinical setting, usually by clinicians, with patients as the subjects of study. It uses the information from classic epidemiology to aid decision making about identified cases of disease.

Clinical trial A prospective study that involves human subjects, designed to determine the effectiveness of a treatment, a surgical procedure, or a therapeutic regimen administered to patients with a specific disease. Clinical trials have four phases:

Phase I Safety and pharmacologic profiles. This involves the initial introduction of a candidate vaccine or drug into a human population to determine its safety and mode of action. In drug trials, this phase may include studies of dose and route of administration. Phase I trials usually involve less than 100 healthy volunteers.

Phase II Pilot efficacy studies. This initial trial aims to examine efficacy in about 200 to 500 volunteers. The focus of vaccine trials is immunogenicity, whereas with drugs the focus is on the demonstration of safety and efficacy in comparison with those of other existing regimens. Often, subjects are randomly allocated to study and control groups.

Phase III Extensive clinical trial. This phase aims to complete assessment of safety and efficacy. It involves large numbers, possibly thousands, of volunteers from one center or many centers (a multicenter trial), usually with random allocation to study and control groups.

Phase IV This phase is conducted after the national drug registration authority (the Food and Drug Administration in the United States) has approved the drug for distribution or marketing. The trial is designed to determine a specific pharmacological effect or the effects of long-term use or to establish the incidence of adverse reactions. Ethical review is required in phase IV trials.

Clinical versus statistical significance The distinction between results in terms of their possible clinical importance rather than simply in terms of their statistical significance. For example, very small differences that have little or no clinical importance may turn out to be statistically significant. The implications of any finding in a medical investigation must be judged on both clinical and statistical grounds.

Clinimetrics The study of indices and rating scales used to describe or measure symptoms, physical signs, and other clinical phenomena in clinical medicine.

Closed sequential design See *sequential analysis*.

Cluster analysis A set of statistical methods for constructing a sensible and informative classification of an initially unclassified set of data using the variable values observed on each individual or item.

Cluster sampling A sampling method in which each unit (cluster) selected is a group of persons (all persons in a city block, a family, a school, or a hospital) rather than an individual.

Code of conduct A formal statement of desirable conduct that research workers or practitioners are expected to honor. Examples are the Hippocratic Oath, the Nuremberg Code, and the Helsinki Declaration.

Coefficient of concordance A measure of the agreement among several rankings or categories.

Coefficient of determination The square of the correlation coefficient between two variables. It gives the proportion of the variation in one variable that is accounted for by the other.

Coefficient of variation A measure of spread for a set of data, defined as 100 x standard deviation / mean. Originally proposed as a way of comparing the variability in different distributions but found to be sensitive to errors in the mean.

Collinearity Very high correlation between variables. See *multicollinearity.*

Comorbidity A disease(s) that coexist(s) in a study participant in addition to the index condition that is the subject of study.

Conditional probability The probability that event *A* occurs given the outcome of some other event, event *B*; usually written $P(A|B)$. Conditional probabilities obey all the axioms of probability theory. See *Bayes's theorem.*

Confidence interval The computed interval with a given probability, e.g., 95 percent, that the true value of a variable such as a mean, proportion, or rate is contained within the interval.

Confidence limits The upper and lower boundaries of the confidence interval.

Confidence profile method A method of meta-analysis that uses a set of quantitative techniques that include parameters, functions, and prior distributions (in a Bayesian application). Its goal is to use evidence to derive maximum likelihood estimates and covariances (in a non-Bayesian application) or joint probability distributions (in a Bayesian application) for parameters of interest. Distributions and estimates can be used to make decisions about interventions or calculations of other parameters or to plan research to gather additional information about any parameter.

Confounding A process observed in some factorial designs in which a measure of the effect of an exposure on risk is distorted because of the association of the exposure with some other factor(s) that influences the outcome under study.

Confounding variable A variable that can cause or prevent the outcome of interest, is not an intermediate variable, and is associated with the factor under investigation.

Contingency table A tabular cross-classification of data such that subcategories of one characteristic are indicated horizontally (in rows) and subcategories of another characteristic are indicated vertically (in columns). The simplest contingency table is the fourfold or two-by-two table analyzed by using the chi-square statistic. Three- and higher-dimensional tables are analyzed by using log-linear models.

Continual reassessment method An approach that applies Bayesian inference to determine the maximum tolerated dose in a phase I trial. The method begins by assuming a logistic regression model for the dose-toxicity relationship and a prior distribution for the parameters. After each patient's toxicity result becomes available, the posterior distribution of the parameters is recomputed and used to estimate the probability of toxicity at each of a series of dose levels.

Control group Subjects with whom comparison is made in a case-control study, randomized controlled trial, or some other variety of epidemiological study.

Controlled trial A phase III clinical trial in which an experimental treatment is compared with a control treatment, the latter being either the current standard treatment or a placebo.

Control statistics Statistics calculated from sample values $X_1, X_2, \ldots, X_n$ that elicit information about some characteristic of a process that is being monitored.

Correlation The degree to which variables change together.

Correlation coefficient An index that quantifies the linear relationship between a pair of variables. The coefficient takes values between –1 and 1, with the sign indicating the direction of the relationship and the numerical magnitude indicating its strength. A value of zero indicates the lack of any linear relationship between two variables.

Correlation matrix A square, symmetric matrix with rows and columns corresponding to variables in which the off-diagonal elements are correlations between pairs of variables and the elements on the main diagonal are unity.

Cost-benefit analysis An economic analysis in which the costs of medical care and the benefits of reduced loss of net earnings due to the prevention of premature death or disability are considered. The general rule for the allocation of funds in a cost-benefit analysis is that the ratio of marginal benefit (the benefit of preventing an additional case) to marginal cost (the cost of preventing an additional case) should be equal to or greater than 1.

Cox's proportional hazards model A method that allows the hazard function to be modeled on a set of explanatory variables without making restrictive assumptions about the dependence of the hazard function on time. Estimates of the parameters in the model, i.e., $\beta_1, \beta_2, \ldots, \beta_p$, are usually obtained by maximum likelihood estimation and depend only on the order in which events occur, not on the exact time of their occurrences.

Critical region The values of a test statistic that lead to rejection of a null hypothesis. The size of the critical region is the probability of obtaining an outcome belonging to this region when the null hypothesis is true, i.e., the probability of a Type I error. See also *acceptance region.*

Critical value The value with which a statistic calculated from sample data is compared to determine whether a null hypothesis should be rejected. The value is related to the particular significance level chosen.

Cross-validation The division of data into two subsets of approximately equal size, one of which is used to estimate the parameters in some model of interest and the other of which is used to assess whether the model with these parameter values fits adequately.

Cumulative frequency distribution A listing of the sample values of a variable together with the proportion of the observations less than or equal to each value.

Decision analysis An approach that involves identification of all available choices and the potential outcomes of each in a series of decisions that must be made about aspects of patient care: diagnostic procedures, therapeutic regimens, and prognostic expectations. The range of choices can be plotted on a decision tree, where at each branch or decision node the probabilities of each outcome are displayed.

Decision function A concept used in decision analysis that tells the experimenter how to conduct the statistical aspects of an experiment and what action to take for each possible outcome. See also *loss function.*

Decision tree A graphical representation of the alternatives available at each stage in the process of decision making, where decision options are represented as branches and subsequent possible outcomes are represented as further branches. The decisions and the eventualities are presented in the order in which they are likely to occur. The junction at which a decision must be taken is called a "decision node."

Degrees of freedom (df) The number of independent units of information in a sample relevant to the estimation of a parameter or calculation of a statistic. For example, in a contingency table it is one less than the number of row categories multiplied by one less than the number of column categories. Also used to refer to a parameter of various families of distributions, such as chi-square, Student's t, and F distributions.

Dependent variable A variable whose value is dependent on the effect of another variable(s)—an independent variable(s)—in the relationship under study. In statistics, it is the variable predicted by a regression equation.

Descriptive statistics A general term for methods of summarizing and tabulating data that make their main features more transparent, for example, calculating means and variances and plotting histograms.

Deviance A measure of the extent to which a particular model differs from the saturated model for a data set.

Dichotomous variable Synonym for *binary variable.*

Directionality The direction of inference of a study, i.e., retrospective or prospective, or of the relationship between variables, such as a negative or a positive association indicated by a correlation coefficient.

Discrete variables Variables having only integer values, e.g., number of births or number of pregnancies.

Discriminant analysis A statistical analytical technique used on multivariate data that aims to assess whether or not a set of variables distinguish or discriminate between two (or more) groups of individuals. It separates sets of observed values and allocates new values from two (or more) discrete populations to the correct population with minimal probability of classification.

Distribution The complete summary of the frequencies of the values or categories of a measurement obtained for a group of persons. It tells either how many or what proportion of the group was found to have each value (or each range of values) out of all the possible values that the quantitative measure can have.

Distribution function A function that gives the relative frequency with which a random variable falls at or below each of a series of values. Examples include normal distribution, lognormal distribution, chi-square distribution, t distribution, F distribution, and binomial distribution.

Dose-ranging trial A clinical trial, usually undertaken at a late stage in the development of a drug, to obtain information about the appropriate magnitude of initial and subsequent doses. Most common is the parallel-dose design, in which one group of subjects is given a placebo and other groups are given different doses of the active treatment.

Dose-response curve A plot of the values of a response variable against the corresponding values of the dose of drug received or level of exposure endured.

Dose-response relationship A relationship in which a change in amount, intensity, or duration of exposure is associated with a change—either an increase or a decrease—in the risk of a specified outcome.

Double-blind trial A procedure of blind assignment to study and control groups and blind assessment of outcome, designed to ensure that ascertainment of outcome is not biased by knowledge of the group to which an individual was assigned. Double refers to both subjects or patients and observers or clinicians.

Dummy variables The variables resulting from recording of categorical variables with more than two categories into a series of binary variables.

Effect measure A quantity that measures the effect of a factor on the frequency or risk of health outcome. Three such measures are attributable fractions, which measure the fraction of cases due to a factor; risk and rate differences, which measure the amount a factor adds to the risk or rate of a disease; and risk and rate ratios, which measure the amount by which a factor multiplies the risk or rate of disease.

Effect modifier A factor that modifies the effect of a putative causal factor under study. For example, age is an effect modifier for many conditions, and immunization status is an effect modifier for the consequences of exposure to pathogenic organisms. Effect modification is detected by varying the selected effect measure for the factor under study across levels of another factor.

Efficacy The effect of a treatment relative to the effect a control treatment in the ideal situation in which all persons fully comply with the treatment regimen to which they were assigned by random allocation.

Endpoint A clearly defined outcome or event associated with an individual in a medical investigation. An example is the eath of a patient.

Equipoise A state of genuine uncertainty about the benefits or harms that may result from each of two or more regimens. A state of equipoise is an indication for a randomized controlled trial because there are no ethical concerns about one regimen being better for a particular patient.

Error, Type I (α error) The error of rejecting a true null hypothesis, i.e., declaring that a difference exists when it does not.

Error, Type II (β error) The error of failing to reject a false null hypothesis, i.e., declaring that a difference does not exist when in fact it does.

Estimate Either a single number (point estimate) or a range of numbers (interval estimate) which is inferred to be plausible for some parameter of interest.

Estimation The process of providing a numerical value for a population parameter on the basis of information collected from a sample. If a single figure for the unknown parameter is calculated, the process is called "point estimation." If an interval within which the parameter is likely to fall is calculated, the procedure is called "interval estimation."

Exact method A statistical method based on the actual, i.e., "exact," probability distribution of the study data rather than on an approximation such as the normal or chi-square distribution, e.g., Fisher's exact test.

Experimental study A study in which conditions are under the direct control of the investigator. A population is selected for a planned trial of a regimen whose effects are measured by comparing the outcome of the regimen in the experimental group with the outcome of another regimen in a control group. Clinical trials fall under this heading.

Explanatory trial A clinical trial designed to explain how a treatment works.

Factor A term that is used in a variety of ways in statistics but that is most commonly used to refer to a categorical variable, with a smaller number of levels, under investigation in an experiment as a possible source of variation.

Factor analysis A set of statistical methods for analysis of the correlations among several variables to estimate the number of fundamental dimensions that underlie the observed data and to describe and measure those dimensions.

Factorial design A method of setting up an experiment or study to ensure that all levels of each intervention or classificatory factor occur with all levels of the others and that their possible interactions are investigated. The simplest factorial design is one in which each of two treatments or interventions is either present or absent so that subjects are divided into four groups: those receiving neither treatment, those receiving only the first treatment, those receiving only the second treatment, and those receiving both treatments.

False-negative rate The proportion of cases in which a diagnostic test indicates that a disease is absent from patients who have the disease.

False-positive rate The proportion of cases in which a diagnostic test indicates that a disease is present in disease-free patients.

F distribution The probability distribution of the ratio of two independent random variables, each having a chi-square distribution, divided by their respective degrees of freedom.

Fibonacci dose escalation scheme A scheme designed to estimate the maximum tolerated dose during a phase I clinical trial, using as few patients as possible. Using the National Cancer Institute standards for adverse drug reactions, the procedure begins patient accrual with three patients at an initial dose level and continues at each subsequent dose level until at least one toxicity of grade 3 or above is encountered. Once the latter occurs, three additional patients are entered at that level and six patients are entered into each succeeding level. The search scheme stops when at least two of six patients have toxicities of grade >3.

Fisher's exact test The test for association in a two-by-two table that is based upon the exact hypergeometric distribution of the frequencies within the table. The procedure consists of evaluating the sum of the probabilities associated with the observed table and all possible two-by-two tables that have the same row and column totals as the observed data.

Fisher's information matrix The inverse of the variance-covariance matrix of a set of parameters.

Fisher's z transformation A transformation of Pearson's product moment correlation coefficient, r, given by

$$Z = \frac{1}{2}\log\frac{1+r}{1-r}$$

The statistic z has mean $\frac{1}{2}\log\frac{1+p}{1-p}$, where p is the population correlation value, and variance $\frac{1}{n-3}$, where n is the sample size. The transformation may be used to test hypotheses and to construct confidence intervals for p.

Fishing expedition A term used to describe comparisons made within a data set not specifically prescribed before the start of the study.

Fitted value Refers to the value of the response variable predicted by some estimated model.

Five-number summary A method of summarizing a set of observations by using the minimum value, the lower quartile, the median, upper quartile, and maximum value. Forms the basis of the box-and-whisker plot.

Fixed effects The effects attributable to a finite set of levels of a factor that are of specific interest. For example, the investigator may wish to compare the effects of three particular drugs on a response variable.

Fixed effects model A model that contains only factors with fixed effects.

Frequency distribution See *distribution.*

***F* test** A test for the equality of the variances of two populations having normal distributions, based on the ratio of the variances of a sample of observations taken from each. Commonly used in the analysis of variance, in which testing of whether particular variances are the same also tests for the equality of a set of means.

Function A quality, trait, or fact that is so related to another as to be dependent upon and to vary with this other.

Functional relationship The relationship between the true values of variables, i.e., the values obtained under the assumption that the variables were measured without error.

Funnel plot A plotting device used in meta-analysis to detect publication bias. The estimate of risk is plotted against sample size. If there is no publication bias, the plot is funnel-shaped. Publication bias, in which studies with significant results are more likely to be published than those with small or no significant effects, removes part of the lower left hand corner of the funnel.

Gaussian distribution A bell-shaped frequency distribution of infinite range of a random variable. All possible values of the variable are displayed on the horizontal axis. The frequency (probability) of each value is displayed on the vertical axis, producing the graph of the distribution. The properties are as follows: (1) it is a continuous, symmetrical distribution; both tails extend to infinity; (2) the arithmetic mean, mode, and median are identical; and (3) its shape is completely determined by the mean and standard deviation. Another name for *normal distribution.*

Generalized linear models (GLMs) A class of models that arise from a natural generalization of ordinary linear regression. The function of the expected value of the response variable, y, is modeled as a linear combination of the explanatory variables, $X_1, X_2, \ldots, .X_q$. The other components of such models are a specification of the form of the variance of the response variable and of its probability distribution.

Goodness-of-fit Degree of agreement between an empirically observed distribution and a mathematical or rhetorical distribution.

Goodness-of-fit statistics Measures of the agreement between a set of sample observations and the corresponding values predicted from some model of interest. Examples are chi-square statistic, deviance, and likelihood ratio.

Group sequential design See *sequential analysis.*

Half-normal plot A plot for diagnosing model inadequacy or revealing the presence of outliers, in which the absolute values of, e.g., the residuals from a multiple regression are plotted against the quantiles of the standard normal distribution. Outliers will appear at the top right of the plot as points that are separated from the others, whereas systematic departures from a straight line could indicate that the model is unsatisfactory.

Hazard function The probability that an individual experiences an event (death, improvement, etc.) in a small time interval, given that the individual has survived up to the beginning of the interval. It is a measure of how likely an individual is to experience an event as a function of the age of the individual. The hazard function may remain constant, increase, or decrease. See also *survival function* and *bathtub curve.*

Hazard rate A theoretical measure of the risk of occurrence of an event, e.g., death or a new disease, at a point in time, t, defined mathematically as the limit, as Δt approaches zero, or of the probability that an individual well at time t will experience the event by $t + \Delta t$, divided by Δt.

Hazard regression A procedure for modeling the hazard rate that does not depend on the assumptions made in Cox's proportional hazards model, namely, that the loghazard function is an additive function of both time and the vector of covariates.

Heteroscedasticity Nonconstancy of the variance of a measure over the levels of the factors under study.

Histogram A graphical representation of a set of observations, in which class frequencies are represented by the areas of rectangles centered on the class interval.

Homoscedasticity Constancy of the variance of a measure over the levels of the factors under study.

Human immunodeficiency virus (HIV) The pathogenic organism responsible for acquired immunodeficiency syndrome (AIDS).

Human leukocyte antigen (HLA) Antigens on cell surfaces that are important for foreign antigen recognition and that play a role in the coordination and activation of the immune response.

Hypergeometric distribution The exact probability distribution of the frequencies in a two-by-two contingency table, conditional on the marginal frequencies being fixed at their observed levels. Usually approximated by the binomial distribution.

Independent variable One of (perhaps) several variables that appear as arguments in a regression equation.

Indicator variable A variable that takes only one of two possible values, with one (usually 1) indicating the presence of a condition and the other (usually 0) indicating the absence of the condition. Used mainly in *regression analysis.*

Informative censoring Censored observations that occur for reasons related to treatment, e.g., when treatment is withdrawn as a result of a deterioration in the physical condition of a patient.

Informative prior A term used in the context of Bayesian inference to indicate a prior distribution that reflects empirical or theoretical information regarding the value of an unknown parameter.

Informed consent The voluntary consent given by a patient to participate in, usually, a clinical trial after being informed of its purpose, method of treatment, procedure for assignment to treatment, benefits and risks associated with participation, and required data collection procedures and schedule.

Initial data analysis The first phase in the examination of a data set that consists of a number of informal steps, including checking the quality of the data, calculating simple summary statistics, and constructing appropriate graphs. The general aim is to clarify the structure of the data, obtain a simple descriptive summary, and possibly get ideas for a more sophisticated analysis.

Instantaneous death rate Synonym for *hazard function.*

Intention-to-treat analysis A procedure in which all patients randomly allocated to a treatment in a clinical trial are analyzed together as representing that treatment, whether or not they received or completed the prescribed regimen. Failure to follow this step defeats the main purpose of random allocation and can invalidate the results.

Interaction The interdependent operation of two or more causes to produce or prevent an effect.

Interim analysis Analysis made before the planned end of a clinical trial, usually with the aim of detecting treatment differences at an early stage and thus preventing as many patients as possible from receiving an "inferior" treatment.

Intermediate variable (intervening or mediator variable) A variable that occurs in a causal pathway from an independent to a dependent variable. It causes variation in the dependent variable and is caused to vary by the independent variable. Its value is altered to block or alter the effect(s) of another factor. Such a variable is statistically associated with both the independent and the dependent variables.

Interquartile range A measure of spread given by the difference between the first and third quartiles of a sample.

Interrupted time series design A study in which a single group of subjects is measured several times before and after some event or manipulation. Also used to describe investigation of a single subject. See n-*of-1 clinical trials*.

Interval censored observations Observations that often arise in the context of studies of time elapsed to a particular event when subjects are not monitored continuously. Instead, the prior occurrence of the event of interest is detectable only at specific times of observation, e.g., at the time of medical examination.

Intervention study An investigation involving intentional change in some aspect of the status of the subjects, e.g., introduction of a preventive or therapeutic regimen, to test a hypothesis. Usually it is an experiment such as a randomized clinical trial.

Iterated bootstrap A two-stage procedure in which the samples from the original bootstrap population are themselves bootstrapped. The technique can give confidence intervals of more accurate coverage than simple bootstrapping.

Iteration The successive repetition of a mathematical process, using the result of one stage as the input for the next.

Jackknife A technique for estimating the variance and the bias of an estimator. If the sample size is n, the estimator is applied to each subsample of size $n - 1$, obtained by dropping a measurement from analysis. The sum of squared differences between each of the resulting estimates and their mean, multiplied by $(n - 1)/n$, is the jackknife estimate of variance; the difference between the mean and the original estimate, multiplied by $(n - 1)$, is the jackknife estimate of bias.

Kaplan-Meier estimate A nonparametric method of compiling life or survival tables. This combines calculated probabilities of survival and estimates to allow censored observations, which are assumed to occur randomly. The intervals are defined as ending each time that an event, (e.g., death or withdrawal) occurs and are therefore unequal.

Kappa coefficient A chance corrected index of the agreement between, e.g., judgments and diagnoses made by two raters. Calculated as the ratio of the observed excess over chance agreement to the maximum possible excess over chance, the coefficient takes the value unity when there is perfect agreement and the value zero when observed agreement is equal to chance agreement.

Kendall's tau statistic Measures of the correlation between two sets of rankings. Kendall's tau statistic is a rank correlation coefficient based on the number of inversions in one ranking compared with the number of inversions in another, e.g., on S, given by $S = P - Q$, where P is the number of concordant pairs of observations, that is, pairs of observations such that their rankings on the two variables are in the same direction, and Q is the number of discordant pairs for which rankings on the two variables are in the reverse direction.

Kruskal-Wallis test A distribution-free method that is the analogue of the analysis of variance of a one-way design. It tests whether the groups to be compared have the same population median.

Kurtosis The extent to which the peak of a unimodal probability distribution or frequency distribution departs from the shape of a normal distribution by either being more pointed (leptokurtic) or flatter (platykurtic). For a normal distribution, the value of kurtosis is zero (mesokurtic).

Least significant difference test An approach to comparing a set of means that controls the familywise error rate at some particular level, say α. The hypothesis of the equality of the means is tested first by an α-level F test. If this test is not significant, then the procedure terminates without making detailed inferences on pairwise differences; otherwise, each pairwise difference is tested by an α-level Student's t test.

Least squares estimation A method used to estimate parameters, particularly in regression analysis, by minimizing the difference between the observed response and the value predicted by the model. Often referred to as "ordinary least squares" to differentiate this simple version of the technique from more involved versions, such as weighted least squares and iteratively weighted least squares.

Likelihood distance test A procedure for the detection of outliers that uses the difference between the log likelihood of the complete data set and the log likelihood when a particular observation is removed. If the difference is large, then the observation involved is considered an outlier.

Likelihood function A function constructed from a statistical model and a set of observed data that gives the probability of the observed data for various values of the unknown model parameters. The parameter values that maximize the probability are the maximum likelihood estimates of the parameters.

Likelihood ratio The ratio of the likelihoods of the data under two hypotheses, H_0 and H_1. May be used to assess H_0 against H_1.

Likert scales An ordinal scale of responses to a question or statement ordered in a hierarchical sequence, such as from "strongly agree" through "no opinion" to "strongly disagree."

Linear function A function of a set of variables, parameters, etc., that does not contain powers or cross-products quantities.

Linear model A statistical model in which the expected value of a parameter for a given value of a factor, x, which is assumed to be equal to $a + bx$, where a and b are constants.

Linear regression Regression analysis of data using linear models.

Linear trend A relationship between two variables in which the values of one variable change at a constant rate as the value of the other variable increases.

Linkage analysis A method used to test the hypothesis that a genetic marker of known location is on a chromosome different from that on which a gene postulated to govern susceptibility to a disease is located.

Lods A term often used in epidemiology for the logarithm of an odds ratio. Also used in genetics for the logarithm of a likelihood ratio.

Logarithmic transformation The transformation of a variable, x, obtained by taking $y = \log(x)$. Often used when the frequency distribution of the variable, x, shows a moderate to large degree of skewness to achieve normality.

Logistic regression A form of regression analysis used when the response variable is a binary variable.

Logit The logarithm of the ratio of frequencies of two different categorical outcomes, such as healthy versus sick.

Logit confidence limits The upper and lower ends of the confidence interval for the logarithm of the odds ratio.

Log-linear model A statistical model that uses an analysis of variance type of approach for the modeling of frequency counts in contingency tables.

Log-normal distribution The probability distribution of a variable, x, for which $\log (x - a)$ has a normal distribution with mean m and variance σ^2.

Log-rank test A method for comparing the survival times of two or more groups of subjects that involves the calculation of observed and expected frequencies of failures in separate time intervals.

Loss function A concept used in decision analysis that assigns numerical values to making good or poor decisions.

Low-dose extrapolation The process applied to the results from bioassays for carcinogenicity conducted with animals at doses that are generally well above human exposure levels to assess risk in humans.

Main effect An estimate of the independent effect of (usually) a factor variable on a response variable in an analysis of variance.

Mann-Whitney test A test that compares two groups of ordinal scores and that shows the probability that they form parts of the same distribution. It is a nonparametric equivalent of the *t* test.

Mantel-Haenszel estimate An estimate of the assumed common odds ratio in a series of two-by-two contingency tables arising from different populations, e.g., occupation or country of origin.

Mantel-Haenszel test A calculated test statistic that uses a standard normal deviate rather than a chi-square value. The test, used to control for confounding, examines the null hypothesis that the variables are independent by looking at just one of the four cells.

Mantel's trend test A regression test of the odds ratio against a numerical variable representing ordered categories of exposure. It may be used to analyze the results of a case-control study.

Markov process A stochastic process such that the conditional probability distribution for the state at any future instant, given the present state, is unaffected by any additional knowledge of the past history of the system. See also *random walk*.

Masking Procedure intended to keep a participant(s) in a study from knowing some fact(s) or observation(s) that might bias or influence that participant's actions or decisions regarding the study. See also *blinding*.

Matching The process of making a study group and a comparison group comparable with respect to extraneous factors. Often used when selecting cases and controls in retrospective studies to control variation in a response variable due to sources other than those immediately under investigation.

Maximum likelihood estimate (MLE) The value for an unknown parameter that maximizes the probability of obtaining exactly the data that were observed.

Maximum tolerated dose The highest possible dose of a drug that can be given with acceptable toxicity to the patient. This dose is usually determined in a phase I clinical trial and is the dose recommended for use in future studies.

McNemar's test A form of the chi-square test for matched-pairs data. It is a special case of the Mantel-Haenszel test.

Mean squared error The expected value of the square of the difference between an estimator and the true value of a parameter. If the estimator is unbiased, then the mean squared error is simply the variance of the estimator. For a biased estimator the mean squared error is equal to the sum of the variance and the square of the bias.

Mean square ratio The ratio of two mean squares in analysis of variance.

Mean squares The name used in the context of analysis of variance for estimators of particular variances of interest. For example, in the analysis of a one-way design, the within-groups mean square estimates the assumed common variance in *k* groups.

Measurement bias Systematic error arising from inaccurate measurements (or classification) of a study variable(s) for subjects.

Measurement error Errors in reading, calculating, or recording a numerical value. The difference between the observed values of a variable recorded under similar conditions and some fixed true value.

Measurement scale The range of possible values for a measurement, e.g. the set of possible responses to a question.

Measures of association Numerical indices quantifying the strength of the statistical dependence of two or more qualitative variables.

Median A measure of central tendency. It is the value in a set of ranked observations that divides the data into two parts of equal size. When there is an odd number of observations, the median is the middle value. When there is an even number of observations, the median is calculated as the average of the two central values.

Meta-analysis The process of using statistical methods to combine the results of two or more independent studies to yield an overall answer to a question of interest. The rationale behind this approach is to provide a test with more power than that provided by the separate studies themselves.

Minimization A method for allocation of patients to treatments in clinical trials that is usually an acceptable alternative to random allocation. The procedure ensures balance between the groups to be compared on prognostic variables, by allocating with a high degree of probability the next patient to enter the trial to whatever treatment would minimize the overall imbalance between the groups on the prognostic variables, at that stage of the trial.

Minimum chi-squared estimation A method of estimation that finds estimates of the parameters of some model of interest by minimizing the chi-squared statistic for the assessment of differences between the observed values and those predicted by the model.

Missing values Observations missing from a set of data. These occur for a variety of reasons, e.g., subjects drop out of the study, subjects do not appear for one or other of the scheduled visits, or there is an equipment failure. Otherwise known as "missing completely at random."

Mixed-effects model A model usually encountered in the analysis of longitudinal data in which some of the parameters are considered to have fixed effects and some are considered to have random effects. For example, in a clinical trial with two treatment groups in which the response variable is recorded for each subject at a number of visits, the treatments would usually be regarded as having fixed effects and the subjects would usually be regarded as having random efffects.

Mode One of the measures of central tendency. It is the most frequently occurring value in a set of observations.

Monte Carlo method Method for finding solutions to mathematical and statistical problems by simulation.

Multicenter study A clinical trial conducted simultaneously in a number of participating hospitals or clinics, with all centers following a universal study protocol and with independent random allocation within each center.

Multicollinearity In multiple regression analysis, a situation in which at least some of the independent variables are highly correlated directly or indirectly with each other. Such a situation can result in inaccurate estimates of the parameters in the regression model.

Multilevel analysis Method of analysis that explains individual outcomes in terms of both individual and environmental or aggregate variables.

Multimodal distribution A probability distribution or frequency distribution with several modes. Multimodality is often taken as an indication that the observed distribution results from the mixing of the distributions of relatively distinct groups of observations.

Multinomial distribution The probability distribution associated with the classification of each of a sample of individuals into one of several mutually exclusive and exhaustive categories. When the number of categories is two, the distribution is called binomial.

Multiple comparison tests Procedures for detailed simultaneous examination of the differences between a set of means, usually after a general hypothesis that they are all equal has been rejected. Examples are Bonferroni correction, Duncan's multiple-range test, Dunnett's test, and Tukey's method. No single technique is best in all situations, and a major distinction between techniques is how they control the possible inflation of the Type I error.

Multiple correlation coefficient The correlation between the observed values of the dependent variable in a multiple regression and the values predicted by the estimated regression equation. Often used as an indicator of how useful the explanatory variables are in predicting the response.

Multiple end points A term used to describe the variety of outcome measures used in many clinical trials. There are a number of ways to measure treatment success, e.g, length of patient survival, percentage of patients experiencing tumor regression, or percentage of patients surviving for 2 years. The aim in using a variety of such measures is to gain better knowledge of the differences between the treatments being compared.

Multiple regression A statistical model in which a continuous response variable, y, is regressed on a number of explanatory variables, $X_1, X_2, \ldots, X_q$. The model is

$$E(y) = \beta_0 + \beta_1 X_1 + \ldots + \beta_q X_q$$

where E denotes the expected value. The parameters in the model, the regression coefficients β_0, β_1, β_q, are generally estimated by least squares estimation. Each coefficient gives the change in the response variable corresponding to a unit change in the appropriate explanatory variable, conditional on the other variables remaining constant.

Multiplication rule for probabilities For events A and B that are independent, the probability that both occur is the product of the separate probabilities, i.e., $P(A \text{ and } B) = P(A)\, P(B)$, where P denotes probability.

Multiplicative model A model in which the combined effect of a number of factors, when applied together, is the product of their separate effects.

Multivariate analysis An analytical method that allows the simultaneous study of two or more dependent variables.

Multivariate analysis of variance A procedure for testing the equality of the mean vectors of more than two populations. The technique is analogous to the analysis of variance of univariate data, except that the groups are compared on q response variables simultaneously. In the univariate case, F tests are used to assess the hypotheses of interest. In the multivariate case, no single test statistic that is optimal in all situations can be constructed.

Multivariate data Data for which each observation consists of values for more than one random variable, e.g., measurements of blood pressure, temperature, and heart rate for a number of subjects.

Multivariate distribution The simultaneous probability distribution of a set of random variables.

Multivariate probit analysis A method for assessing the effect of explanatory variables on a set of two or more correlated binary response variables.

Negative predictive value The probability that a person having a negative result or a diagnostic test does not have the disease.

Newman-Keuls test A multiple-comparison test used to investigate in more detail the differences existing between a set of means, as indicated by a significant F test in an analysis of variance.

n-of-1 clinical trial A variation of a randomized controlled trial in which a sequence of alternative treatment regimens is randomly allocated to a single patient. The outcomes of successive regimens are compared, with the aim being determination of the optimum regimen for the patient.

Nominal variable A variable that gives the appropriate label of an observation after allocation to one of several possible categories, for example, gender (male or female), marital status (married, single, or divorced), or blood group (A, B, AB, or O).

Nomogram A line chart showing scales for the variables involved in a particular formula in such a way that corresponding values for each variable lie on a straight line that intersects all the scales.

Nonrandomized clinical trial A trial in which a series of consecutive patients receive a new treatment and those who respond (according to some predefined criterion) continue to receive it. Patients who fail to respond receive an alternative treatment. The two groups are then compared on one or more outcome variables.

Nonresponse A term used for failure to provide the relevant information being collected in a survey for a variety of reasons. A large number of nonrespondents may introduce bias into the final results.

No-observed-effect level (NOEL) The dose level of a compound below which there is no evidence of an effect on the response of interest.

Normal approximation to the binomial distribution A normal distribution with mean np and variance $np(1 - p)$ that acts as an approximation to a binomial distribution as n, the number of trials, increases. The term p represents the probability of a "success" of any trial.

Normal distribution A probability distribution of a random variable, x, that is assumed by many statistical methods. The properties of a normal distribution are as follows: (1) it is a continuous, symmetrical distribution; both tails extend to infinity; (2) the arithmetic mean, mode, and median are identical; and (3) its shape is determined by the mean and standard deviation. Synonym for *Gaussian distribution*.

Null distribution The probability distribution of a test statistic when the null hypothesis is true.

Null hypothesis The statistical hypothesis that one variable has no association with another variable or set of variables or that two or more population distributions do not differ from one another.

Number needed to treat In clinical treatment regimens, the number of patients with a specified condition who must follow the specified regimen for a prescribed period to prevent the occurrence of a specified complication(s) or an adverse outcome(s) of the condition.

O'Brien's two-sample tests Tests that assess the differences between treatment groups and that take account of the possible heterogeneous nature of the response treatment. They may lead to the identification of subgroups of patients for whom the experimental therapy might have the most or the least benefit.

Odds The ratio of the probability of the occurrence of an event to that of the nonoccurrence of the event.

Odds ratio The ratio of the odds for a binary variable in two groups of subjects. For example, if the two possible states of the variable are labeled "success" and "failure," then the odds ratio is a measure of the odds of a success in one group relative to that in the other.

One:*m* matching A form of matching often used when control subjects are more readily obtained than cases. A number, m ($m > 1$), of controls are attached to each case, with these being known as the matched set. The theoretical efficiency of such matching in estimating, e.g., relative risk, is $m/(m+1)$, so one control per case is 50 percent efficient, whereas four controls per case is 80 percent efficient. Increasing the number of controls beyond 5 to 10 brings rapidly diminishing returns.

One-tailed test A statistical significance test based on the assumption that the data have only one possible direction of variability. The choice between a one-sided test and a two-sided test must be made before any test statistic is calculated.

One way design See *analysis of variance.*

Ordinal variable A measurement that allows a sample of individuals to be ranked with respect to some characteristic but for which differences at different points of the scale are not necessarily equivalent. For example, anxiety might be rated on a scale of "none," "mild," "moderate," and "severe," with the values 0, 1, 2, and 3 respectively, being used to label the categories.

Outcomes All the possible results that may stem from exposure to a causal factor or from preventive or therapeutic interventions; all identified changes in health status arising as a consequence of the handling of a health problem.

Outliers Observations that differ so widely from the rest of the data as to lead one to suspect that a gross error may have been committed in measurement or recording.

Overmatching A situation that may arise when the matching procedure partially or completely obscures evidence of a true causal association between the independent and dependent variables. The matching variable may be an intermediate cause in the causal chain, or it may be strongly affected by or a consequence of such an intermediate cause.

Paired availability design A design that can reduce selection bias in situations in which it is not possible to use random allocation of subjects to treatments. In the experimental groups, the new treatment is made available to all subjects, although some may not receive it. In the control groups, the experimental treatment is generally not available to subjects, although some subjects may receive it in special circumstances.

Paired samples In a clinical trial, two samples of observations with the characteristic feature that each observation in one sample has one and only one matching observation in the other sample. One member of each pair receives the experimental regimen, and the other member of each pair receives a suitably designated control regimen.

Parallel groups design A simple experimental setup in which two different groups of patients, e.g., treated and untreated patients, are studied concurrently.

Parallelism in analysis of covariance One of the assumptions made in the analysis of covariance, namely, that the slope of the regression line relating the response variable to the covariate is the same in all treatment groups.

Parametric hypothesis A hypothesis concerning the parameter(s) of a distribution, e.g., the hypothesis that the mean for a population equals the mean for a second population when the populations are each assumed to have a normal distribution.

Parametric methods Procedures for testing hypotheses about parameters in a population described by a specified distributional form, often a normal distribution. Student's t test is an example of such a method.

Partial correlation The correlation between a pair of variables after adjusting for the effect of a third variable.

Partial multiple correlation coefficient An index for examining the linear relationship between a response variable and a group of explanatory variables while controlling for another group of variables.

Path analysis A mode of analysis involving assumptions about the direction of causal relationships between linked sequences and configurations of variables. This allows the analyst to construct and test the appropriateness of alternative models (in the form of a path diagram) of the causal relations that may exist within the array of variables.

Pearson's product moment correlation See *correlation coefficient.*

Person-time A measurement combining persons and time, used as denominator in person-time incidence and mortality rates. It is the sum of individual units of time that the persons in the study population have been exposed to the conditions of interest. The most frequently used person-time is person-years.

Person-time incidence rate A measure of the incidence rate of an event, e.g., disease or death, in a population at risk, given by

$$\frac{\text{number of events occurring during the interval}}{\text{number of person-time units at risk observed during the interval}}$$

Person-years See *person-time.*

Placebo effect A phenomenon in which patients given only inert substances often show subsequent clinical improvement compared with patients who received the actual treatment.

Placebo reactor A term for those patients in a clinical trial who report side effects normally associated with the active treatment while receiving a placebo.

Play-the-winner rule A procedure in clinical trials in which the response to treatment is either positive (a success) or negative (a failure). One of the two treatments is selected at random and used on the first patient; thereafter, the same treatment is used on the next patient whenever the response of the previously treated patient is positive and the other treatment is used whenever the response is negative.

Point estimate See *estimate.*

Poisson distribution A distribution function used to describe the occurrence of rare events or to describe the sampling distribution of isolated counts in a continuum of time or space. This distribution is used to model person-time incidence rates.

Polynomial regression A linear model in which powers and possibly cross-products of explanatory variables are included, e.g., $y = \beta_0 + \beta_1 x + \beta_2 x^2$.

Positive predictive value The probability that a person having a positive result on a diagnostic test actually has a particular disease.

Power The probability of rejecting the null hypothesis when it is false. Power gives a method of discriminating between competing tests of the same hypothesis, with the test with the higher power being preferred. It is also the basis of procedures for estimating the sample size needed to detect an effect of a particular magnitude.

Precision A term applied to the likely spread of estimates of a parameter in a statistical model. Measured by the standard error of the estimator, which can be decreased, and hence precision is increased, by using a larger sample size.

Predictor variables The variables that appear on the right side of the equation defining, e.g., multiple regression or logistic regression, and that aim to predict or explain the response variable.

Prior distribution Probability distribution that summarizes information about a random variable or parameter known or assumed at a given time point before further information about empirical data is obtained. It is used in the context of *Bayesian inference.*

Probability The quantitative expression of the chance that an event will occur. It can be defined in a variety of ways, of which the most common is

$$p(A) = \frac{\text{number of times } A \text{ occurs}}{\text{number of times } A \text{ could occur}}$$

Probability distribution For a discrete random variable, a mathematical formula that gives the probability of each value of the variable. Examples are binomial distribution and Poisson distribution. For a continuous random variable, a curve described by a mathematical formula that specifies, by way of areas under the curve, the probability that the variable falls within a particular interval. Examples are normal distribution and exponential distribution.

Probability sample A sample obtained by a method in which every individual in a finite population has a known, but not necessarily equal, chance of being included in the sample.

Probability (p) value The probability of the observed data (or data showing a more extreme departure from the null hypothesis) when the null hypothesis is true.

Probit analysis A technique most commonly used in bioassays, particularly toxilogical experiments in which sets of animals are subject to known levels of a toxin, and a model is required to relate the proportions surviving at a particular dose to the dose. In this type of analysis the probit transformation of a proportion is modeled as a linear function of the dose or, more commonly, the logarithm of the dose. Estimates of the parameters in the models are found by maximum likelihood estimation.

Probit transformation A transformation used in the analysis of dose-response curve.

Proportional hazards model See *Cox's proportional hazards model.*

Proportional odds model A model for investigating the dependence of an ordinal variable on a set of explanatory variables. In the most commonly used version of the model, the cumulative probabilities, $P(y \leq k)$, where y is the response variable with categories $1 \leq 2 \leq 3 \ldots \leq c$, are modeled as linear functions of the explanatory variables via the logistic transformation. The name proportional odds arises since the odds ratio of having a score of k or less for two different sets of values of the explanatory variables does not depend on k.

Protective efficacy (PE) of a vaccine The proportion of cases of disease prevented by the vaccine, usually estimated as PE = (ARU – ARV)/ARU, where ARV and ARU are the attack rates of the disease under study among the vaccinated and unvaccinated cohorts, respectively. For example, if the rate of disease is 100 per 10,000 in an unvaccinated group but only 30 per 10,000 in a comparable vaccinated group, the PE is 70 percent.

Protocol A formal document outlining the proposed procedures for carrying out a clinical trial. The main features of the document are study objectives, patient selection criteria, treatment schedules, methods of patient evaluation, trial design, procedures for dealing with protocol violations, and plans for statistical analysis.

Protocol violations Deliberate or accidental failure of patients to follow one or other aspects of a protocol for a clinical trial. For example, the patients may not have taken their prescribed medication. Such patients are said to show noncompliance.

Quadrant sampling A sampling procedure used with spatial data in which sample areas (the quadrants) are taken and the number of objects or events of interest occurring in each is recorded.

Quantile-quantile (Q-Q) plot An informal method for assessing assumptions when fitting statistical models or using significance tests. For example, in investigating the assumption that a set of data is from a normal distribution, the ordered sample values, $X_{(1)}, X_{(2)}, \ldots X_{(n)}$ are plotted against the values

$\Phi^{-1}(p_i)$

where $p_i = (i - 1/2)/n$, and

$$\Phi(x) = \int_{-\infty}^{x} \frac{1}{\sqrt{2\pi}} e^{-\frac{1}{2}u^2} du.$$

Quantiles Divisions of a probability distribution or frequency distribution into equal, ordered subgroups, e.g., quartiles or percentiles.

Quantit model A three-parameter nonlinear logistic regression model.

Quartiles The values that divide a frequency distribution or probability distribution into four equal parts.

Quasilikelihood A function that is used as the basis for the estimation of parameters when it is not possible (or desirable) to make a particular distributional assumption about the observations, with the consequence that it is not possible to write down their likelihood. The function depends on the assumed relationship between the mean and the variance of the observations.

Quintiles The set of four variate values that divide a frequency distribution or a probability distribution into five equal parts.

Quota sample A sample in which the units are not selected completely at random, but are selected in terms of a certain number of units in each of a number of categories, e.g., 10 men over age 40 or 25 women between ages 30 and 35.

Radial plot of odds ratios A diagram used to display the odds ratios calculated from a number of different clinical trials of the same treatment(s). The diagram consists of a plot of $y = \hat{\Delta}/SE(\hat{\Delta})$ against $x = 1/SE(\hat{\Delta})$, where $\hat{\Delta}$ is the logarithm of the odds ratio from a particular study and *SE* is standard error. Often useful in meta-analysis.

Random allocation, randomization Allocation of individuals to groups, e.g., for experimental and control regimens, by chance. It follows a predetermined plan that is usually devised with the aid of a table of random numbers. The control and experimental groups should be similar at the start of the investigation, and the investigator's personal judgment and prejudices should not influence allocation.

Random effects The effects attributable to an infinite set of levels of a factor, only a randomsample of which occurs in the data.

Randomization tests Procedures for determining statistical significance directly from data, without recourse to some particular sampling distribution. The data are divided repeatedly between treatments, and for each division the relevant test statistic e.g., t or F is calculated to determine the proportion of the data permutations that provide as large a test statistic as that associated with the observed data. If that proportion is smaller than some significance level ?, the results are significant at the ? level.

Randomized clinical trial (RCT) A clinical trial that involves the formation of treatment groups by the process of random allocation.

Randomized consent design A design originally introduced to overcome some of the perceived ethical problems facing clinicians entering patients in randomized clinical trials. After the patient's eligibility is established, the patient is randomized to one of two treatments, treatments A and B. The risks, benefits, and treatment options are discussed with patients randomized to receive treatment A, and the patients are asked if they are willing to receive the therapy. Those who do not agree receive treatment B or some alternative treatment. The same procedure is followed for patients who were randomized to receive treatment B.

Random sample Either a set of n independent and identically distributed random variables or a sample of n individuals selected from a population in such a way that each sample of the same size is equally likely.

Random variable A variable, the values of which occur according to some specified probability distribution.

Random variation The variation in a data set unexplained by identifiable sources.

Random walk The path traversed by a particle that moves in steps, with each step being determined by chance in regard to direction or magnitude, or both. Random walk may be applied to sequential sampling.

Range The difference between the largest and the smallest observations in a data set.

Range of equivalence The range of differences between two treatments being compared in a clinical trial within which it is not possible to make a definite choice of treatment.

Rank correlation coefficients Correlation coefficients that depend only on the ranks of the variables, not on their observed values. Examples are Kendall's tau statistics and Spearman's rho correlation coefficient.

Rank order statistics Statistics based only on the rank of the sample observations, e.g., Kendall's tau statistics.

Rate A measure of the frequency of occurrence of a phenomenon, given by

$$\text{Rate} = \frac{\text{mumber of events in specified period}}{\text{average population during the period}} \times 10^n$$

Ratio The value obtained by dividing one quantity by another: a general term of which rate, proportion, percentage, etc., are subsets. It is an expression of the relationship between a numerator and a denominator in which the two are usually separate and distinct quantities, with neither being included in the other.

Receiver operating characteristic (ROC) curve A plot of the sensitivity (y axis) of a diagnostic test against the complement of its specificity (x axis) that ascertains the balance between specificity and sensitivity corresponding to various cutoffs.

Regression analysis A general term for methods of analysis that are concerned with estimating the parameters in some postulated relationship between a response variable and one or more explanatory variables. Examples are linear regression, logistic regression, and multiple regression.

Regression coefficient, regression weight See *multiple regression.*

Regression diagnostics Procedures designed to investigate the assumptions underlying a regression analysis (e.g., normality or homogeneity of variance) or to examine the influence of particular datum points or small groups of datum points on the estimated regression coefficients.

Regression line Diagrammatic presentation of a regression equation, usually drawn with the independent variable, x, as the abscissa and the dependent variable, y, as ordinate.

Relative risk A measure of the association between exposure to a particular factor and risk of a certain outcome, calculated as

$$\text{Relative risk} = \frac{\text{incidence rate among exposed}}{\text{incidence rate among nonexposed}}$$

Relative survival The ratio of the observed survival for a given group of patients to the survival that group would have experienced on the basis of the life table for the population for which the diagnosis was made.

Reliability The degree to which the results obtained by a measurement procedure can be replicated.

Reproducibility The closeness of results obtained on the same test material under changes of reagents, conditions, techniques, apparatus, laboratories, and so on.

Residual The difference between the observed value of a response variable (yi) and the value predicted by some model of interest (yi). Examination of a set of residuals, usually by informal graphical techniques, allows the assumptions made in the model-fitting exercise (e.g., normality and homogeneity of variance) to be checked.

Residual confounding Potential confounding by factors or variables not yet considered in the analysis, which may be directly observable or not.

Residual sum of squares See *analysis of variance.*

Response bias The systematic component of the difference between information provided by survey respondent and the "truth."

Response rate The number of completed or returned survey instruments (questionnaires, interviews, etc.) divided by the total number of persons who would have been surveyed.

Response variable The variable of primary importance in medical investigations, since the major objective is usually to study the effects of a treatment or other explanatory variables on this variable.

Restricted maximum likelihood estimation (REML) A method of estimation in which estimators of parameters are derived by maximizing the restricted likelihood rather than the likelihood itself.

Resubstitution error rate The estimate of the proportion of subjects misclassified by a rule derived from a discriminant analysis, obtained by reclassifying the training set by using the rule.

Ridge regression A method of regression analysis designed to overcome the possible problem of multicollinearity among the explanatory variables. Such multicollinearity makes it difficult to estimate the separate effects of variables on the response. This form of regression may result in increased precision.

Ridit analysis A method of analysis for ordinal variables that proceeds from the assumption that the ordered categorical scale is an approximation to an underlying, but not directly measurable, continuous variable. Numerical values called ridits are calculated for each category. These values are estimates of the probability that a subject's value on the underlying variable is less than or equal to the midpoint of the corresponding interval.

Risk assessment The qualitative or quantitative estimation of the likelihood of adverse effects that may result from exposure to specified health hazards or from the absence of beneficial influences.

Robust estimation Methods of estimation that work well not only under ideal conditions but also under conditions representing a departure from an assumed distribution or model.

Robust regression A general class of statistical procedures designed to reduce the sensitivity of the parameter estimates to failures in the assumption of the model. For example, least squares estimation is known to be sensitive to outliers, but the impact of such observations can be reduced by basing the estimation process not on a sum-of-squares criterion but on a sum-of-absolute values criterion.

Robust statistics Statistical procedures and tests that work well even when the assumptions on which they are based are moderately violated. An example is Student's *t* test.

Rule of three A method based on the Poisson distribution which states that if in *n* trials zero events of interest are observed, a 95 percent confidence (with limits of 0 and 3) bound on the underlying rate is $3/n$.

Run-in A period of observation before the formation of treatment groups by random allocation, during which subjects acquire experience with the major components of a study protocol. Those subjects who experience difficulty complying with the protocol are excluded, whereas the group of proven compliers is randomized into the trial.

Runs In a series of observations, the occurrence of an uninterrupted sequence of the same value. For example, in the series 1111222433333 there are four "runs", with the single value, 4, being regarded as a run of length unity.

Runs test A test frequently used to detect serial correlations. The test consists of counting the number of runs or sequences of positive and negative residuals and comparing the result with the expected value under the null hypothesis of independence.

Sample size determination The process of deciding, before a study begins, how many subjects should be studied. It takes into account the incidence or prevalence of the condition being studied, the estimated or putative relationship among the variables in the study, the power that is desired, and the allowable Type I error.

Sampling distribution The probability distribution of a statistic. For example, the sampling distribution of the arithmetic mean of samples of size *n*, taken from a normal distribution with mean ? and standard deviation σ, is a normal distribution also with mean ? but with standard deviation $\sigma / \sqrt{n}$.

Sampling error The difference between the sample result and the population characteristic being estimated. In practice, the sampling error can rarely be determined because the population characteristic is not usually known. With appropriate sampling procedures, it can be kept small and the investigator can determine its probable limits of magnitude.

Sampling variation The variation shown by different samples of the same size from the same population.

Sampling zeros Zero frequencies that occur in the cells of contingency tables because of inadequate sample size.

Saturated model A model that contains all main effects and all possible interactions between factors. Such a model contains the same number of parameters as observations and results in a perfect fit for a data set.

Scatter diagram, scattergram, scatterplot A graphic method of displaying the distribution of two variables in relation to each other.

Selection bias The bias that may be introduced into clinical trials and other types of medical investigations whenever a treatment is chosen by the individual involved or is subject to constraints that go unobserved by the researcher.

Semi-interquartile range Half the difference between the upper and lower quartiles.

Sensitivity An index of the performance of a diagnostic test, calculated as the percentage of individuals with a disease who are correctly classified as having the disease, i.e., the conditional probability of having a positive test result given that the disease is present.

Sensitization Administration of antigen to induce a primary immune response.

Sequential analysis A method of analysis in which a statistical test of significance is conducted repeatedly over time as the data are collected. After each observation, the cumulative data are analyzed and one of the following three decisions is taken:

- stop the data collection, reject the null hypothesis, and claim statistical significance;
- stop the data collection, do not reject the null hypothesis, and state that the results are not statistically significant;
- continue the data collection since the accumulated data are inadequate to draw a conclusion.

Three types of sequential analysis are:

- open-ended sequential analysis, used in studies that continue indefinitely until sufficient evidence to reject or fail to reject the null hypothesis has accumulated;
- closed-ended sequential analysis, in which the maximum size of the sample has been set and as data are accumulated and analyzed there is an option to terminate the study before data from the planned sample size have accumulated; and
- group sequential analysis, in which interim analysis is undertaken at planned numbers of intervals, with each interval having accumulated data for a specified number of samples.

Sequential sums of squares A term in regression analysis that refers to the contribution of variables as they are added to the model in a particular sequence. It is the difference in the residual sum of squares before and after adding a variable.

Sickle cell anemia A hereditary, genetically determined hemolytic anemia, one of the hemoglobinopathies, occurring almost exclusively in African Americans, characterized by arthralgia, acute attacks of abdominal pain, ulcerations of the lower extremities, and sickle-shaped erythrocytes in the blood.

Significance level The level of probability at which it is agreed that the null hypothesis will be rejected, conventionally set at 0.05.

Significance test A statistical procedure that, when applied to a set of observations, results in a p value relative to some hypothesis. Examples include Student's t test, z test, and Wilcoxon's signed rank test.

Sign test A test that can be used when combining results of several studies, e.g., in meta-analysis. The test considers the direction of results of individual studies, whether the associations demonstrated are positive or negative.

Similarity coefficient Coefficients that range from zero to unity and that are used to measure the similarity of the variable values of two observations from a set of multivariate data. Most commonly used on binary variables.

Simpson's paradox A form of confounding in which the presence of a confounding variable changes the direction of an association. It may occur in meta-analysis because the sum of the data or results from a number of different studies may be affected by confounding variables that have been excluded by design features from some studies but not others.

Singly censored data Censored observations that occur in clinical trials in which all the patients enter the study at the same time point and in which the study is terminated after a fixed time period.

Skewness The lack of symmetry in a probability distribution.

Spatial data A collection of measurements or observations on one or more variables taken at specified locations and for which the spatial organization of the data is of primary interest.

Specificity An index of the performance of a diagnostic test, calculated as the percentage of individuals without the disease who are classified as not having the disease, i.e., the conditional probability of a negative test result given that the disease is absent.

Square root transformation A transformation of the form $y = \sqrt{x}$, often used to make random variables suspected to have a Poisson distribution more suitable for techniques such as analysis of variance by making their variances independent of their means.

Standard deviation (SD) The most commonly used measure of the spread of a set of observations. Equal to the square root of the variance.

Standard error (SE) The standard deviation of the sampling distribution of a statistic. For example, the standard error of the sample mean of n observations is $\sigma / \sqrt{n}$, where σ^2 is the variance of the original observations.

Standardization A set of techniques used to remove as much as possible the effects of differences in age or other confounding variables when comparing two or more populations. The common method uses weighted averaging of rates specific for age, sex, or some potential confounding variable(s) according to some specified distribution of these variables.

Standard normal distribution A normal distribution with zero mean and unit variance.

Standard normal variable A random variable having a standard normal distribution.

Standard scores Variable values transformed to zero mean and unit variance.

Statistic A numerical characteristic of a sample, e.g., sample mean and sample variance.

Statistical significance An estimate of the probability of the observed or greater degree of association between independent and dependent variables under the null hypothesis. The level of statistical significance is usually stated by the p value.

Statistical test A procedure that is intended to decide whether a hypothesis about the distribution of one or more populations or variables should be rejected or accepted.

Stem-and-leaf plot A method of displaying data resembling a histogram in which each observation is split into two parts, with multiples of 10 along the "stem" and the integers forming the "leaves." The stems are arranged in a column, and the leaves are attached to the relevant stem.

Stochastic process A process that incorporates some element of randomness, in a series of random variables, xt, where t assumes values in a certain range T. In most cases xt is an observation at time t and T is a time range.

Stopping rules Procedures that allow interim or sequential analyses in clinical trials at predefined times and that specify the conditions or criteria under which the trial shall be terminated while preserving the Type I error at some prespecified level.

Stratified logrank test A method for comparing the survival experiences of two groups of subjects given different treatments when the groups are stratified by age or some other prognostic variable.

Stratified randomization A randomization procedure in clinical trials in which strata are identified and subjects are randomly allocated to treatments within each stratum without sacrificing the advantages of random allocation.

Structural zeros Zero frequencies occurring in the cells of contingency tables that arise because it is theoretically impossible for an observation to fall in the cell.

Student's t distribution The probability distribution of the ratio of a standard normal variable to the square root of a variable with a chi-square distribution. The shape of the distribution varies with n, and as n gets larger the shape of the t distribution approaches that of the standard normal distribution.

Student's t tests Significance tests for assessing hypotheses about population means. One version, known as single-sample t test, is used in situations in which it is required to test whether the mean for a population takes a particular value. Another version, known as independent-samples t test, is applied when independent samples are available from each population and is designed to test the equality of the means for the two populations.

Subgroup analysis The analysis of particular subgroups of patients in a clinical trial to assess possible treatment-subgroup interactions. Analysis of many subgroups for treatment effects can increase overall Type I error rates.

Subjective end points End points in clinical trials that can be measured only by subjective clinical rating scales.

Surrogate end point In clinical trials it refers to an outcome measure that an investigator considers to be highly correlated with an endpoint of interest but that can be measured at lower expense or at an earlier time. In some cases, ethical issues may suggest the use of a surrogate endpoint.

Survival function The probability that the survival time of an individual is longer than some particular value. A plot of this probability against time is called a survival curve and is a useful component in the analysis of such data.

Symmetrical distribution A probability distribution or frequency distribution that is symmetrical about some central value.

Systematic allocation Procedures for allocating treatments to patients in a clinical trial that attempts to emulate random allocation by using some systematic scheme, such as giving treatment A to those people with birth dates on even dates and treatment B to those with birth dates on odd days.

Systematic error A term often used in a clinical laboratory to describe the difference in results caused by a bias of an assay.

Target population The collection of individuals, items, measurements, etc., about which it is required to make inferences. At times it is used to indicate the population from which a sample is drawn, and at times it is used to denote any reference population about which inferences are required.

t distribution The distribution of a quotient of independent random variables, the numerator of which is a standardized normal variate and the denominator of which is the positive square root of the quotient of a chi-square-distributed variate and its number of degrees of freedom.

Test statistic A statistic used to assess a particular hypothesis in relation to some population. The essential requirement of such a statistic is a known distribution when the null hypothesis is true.

Tied observations A term usually applied to ordinal variables to indicate observations that take the same value on a variable.

Time-dependent covariates Covariates whose values change over time. Examples are age and weight.

Time-independent covariates Covariates whose values remain constant over time. An example is a pretreatment measurement of some characteristic.

Tmax A measure traditionally used to compare treatments in bioequivalence trials. It is the time at which a patient's highest recorded values occur.

Total sum of squares The sum of the squared deviations of all the observations from their mean.

Trapezium rule A simple rule for approximating the integral of a function, $f(x)$, between two limits.

Treatment allocation ratio The ratio of the number of subjects allocated to the two treatments in a clinical trail. Equal allocation is most common in practice, but it may be advisable to allocate patients randomly in other ratios when a new treatment is compared with an old one, or when one treatment is much more difficult or expensive to administer.

Treatment cross contamination An instance in which a patient assigned to receive a particular treatment in a clinical trial is exposed to one of the other treatments during the course of the trial.

Treatment received analysis Analyzing the results of a clinical trial by the treatment received by a patient rather than by the treatment allocated at randomization as in intent-to-treat analysis.

Treatment trial Synonym for *clinical trial.*

Trend Movement in one direction of the values of a variable over a period of time.

Triple blind A study in which the subjects, observers, and analysts are blinded as to which subjects received what interventions.

Truncated data Data for which sample values larger (truncated on the right) or smaller (truncated on the left) than a fixed value are either not recorded or not observed.

t test Test that uses a statistic that, under the null hypothesis, has the *t* distribution to test whether two means differ significantly or to test linear regression or correlation coefficients.

Tumorigenic dose 50 (TD50) The daily dose of a compound required to halve the probability of remaining tumorless at the end of a standardized lifetime.

Two-armed bandit allocation An allocation procedure for forming treatment groups in a clinical trial in which the probability of assigning a patient to a particular treatment is a function of the observed differences in outcomes for patients already enrolled in the trial.

Two-by-two contingency table A contingency table with two rows and two columns formed from cross classification of two binary variables.

Two-phase sampling A sampling scheme involving two distinct phases: first, information about particular variables of interest is collected for all members of the sample, and second, information about other variables is collected for a subsample of the individuals in the original sample.

Two-stage sampling A procedure most often used in the assessment of quality assurance before, during, and after the manufacture of, e.g., a drug product. This would involve randomly sampling a number of packages of some drug and then sampling a number of tablets from each of these packages.

Two-stage stopping rule A procedure sometimes used in clinical trials in which results are first examined after only a fraction of the planned number of subjects in each group have completed the trial. The relevant test statistic is calculated and the trial is stopped if the difference between the treatments is significant at stage 1 level . Otherwise, additional subjects in each treatment group are recruited, the test statistic is calculated again, and the groups are compared at stage 2 level α_2, where α and α_2 are chosen to give an overall significance level of α.

Two-tailed test A statistical significance test based on the assumption that the data are distributed in both directions from some central value(s).

Type I error The error that results when the null hypothesis is falsely rejected.

Type II error The error that results when the null hypothesis is falsely accepted.

Unanimity rule A requirement that all of a number of diagnostic tests yield positive results before declaring that a patient has a particular complaint.

Unbiased estimator An estimator that for all sample sizes has an expected value equal to the parameter being estimated. If an estimator tends to be unbiased as the sample size increases, it is referred to as "asymptotically unbiased."

Uniform distribution The probability distribution of a random variable having constant probability over an interval. The most commonly encountered uniform distribution is one in which the parameters α and β take the values 0 and 1, respectively.

Unimodal distribution A probability distribution or frequency distribution having only a single mode.

Unit normal variable Synonym for *standard normal variable.*

Univariate data Data involving a single measurement for each subject or patient.

Unweighted means analysis An approach to the analysis of two-way and higher-order factorial designs when there are an unequal number of observations in each cell. The analysis is based on cell means, using the harmonic mean of all cell frequencies as the sample size for all cells.

U-shaped distribution A probability distribution or frequency distribution shaped more or less like a letter U, although not necessarily symmetrical. The distribution has its greatest frequencies at the two extremes of the range of the variable.

Utility In economics, utility means preference for or desirability of a particular outcome.

Utility analysis A method in clinical decision analysis in which the outcome refers to being or becoming healthy rather than sick or disabled.

Vague prior A term used for the prior distribution in Bayesian inference in the situation in which there is complete ignorance about the value of a parameter.

Validity The extent to which a measuring instrument is measuring what was intended.

Validity checks A part of data editing in which one checks that only allowable values or codes are given for the answers to questions asked of subjects.

Validity, measurement An expression of the degree to which a measurement measures what it intends to measure.

Validity, study The degree to which the inference drawn from a study, especially generalizations extending beyond the study sample, are warranted after taking into account the study methods, the representativeness of the study sample, and the nature of the population from which it is drawn.

Variable Any attribute, phenomenon, or event that can have different values from time to time.

Variable, antecedent A variable that causally precedes the association of the outcome under study.

Variable, confounding See *confounding*.

Variable, control Independent variable other than the "hypothetical causal variable" that has a potential effect on the dependent variable and that is subject to control by analysis.

Variable, uncontrolled A (potentially) confounding variable that has not been brought under control by design or analysis.

Variance A measure of the variation shown by a set of observations, defined by the sum of squares of the deviation from the mean divided by the number of degrees of freedom in the set of observations. In a population, the second moment about the mean.

Variance components Variances of random-effect terms in linear models. For example, in a simple mixed model for longitudinal data, both subject effects and error terms are random, and estimation of their variances is of some importance. In the case of a balanced design, estimation of these variances is usually achieved directly from the appropriate analysis of variance table by equating mean squares to their expected values. When the data are unbalanced, a variety of estimation methods might be used, although maximum likelihood estimation and restricted maximum likelihood estimation are most often used.

Variance-covariance matrix A symmetric matrix in which the off-diagonal elements are the covariances (sample or population) of pairs of variables and the elements on the main diagonal are the variances (sample or population) of the variables.

Variance inflation factor An indicator of the effect that the other explanatory variables have on the variance of a regression coefficient of a particular variable, given by the reciprocal of the square of the multiple correlation coefficient of the variable with the remaining variables.

Variance ratio distribution Synonym for *F* distribution.

Variance ratio test Synonym for *F* test.

Variance-stabilizing transformations Transformation designed so that the variance of the transformed variable is independent of parameters.

Vector A matrix having only one row or column.

Venn diagram A graphical representation of the extent to which two or more quantities or concepts are mutually inclusive and mutually exclusive.

Virtually safe dose The exposure level to some toxic agent corresponding to an acceptably small risk of suffering an ill effect. From a regulatory perspective, this typically means an increased risk of no more than 10^{6} or 10^{4} above the background.

Volunteer bias A possible source of bias in clinical trials involving volunteers, but not involving random allocation, because of the known propensity of volunteers to respond better to treatment than other patients.

Wald's test A test for the hypothesis that a vector of parameters, $\theta' = [\theta_1, \theta_2, \ldots, \theta_m]$, is the null vector. The test statistic is,

$$W = \hat{\theta}' V^{-1} \hat{\theta}$$

where $\hat{\theta}'$ contains the estimated parameter values and V is the asymptotic variance-covariance matrix of $\hat{\theta}$. Under the hypothesis, *W* has an asymptotic chi-square distribution with degrees of freedom equal to the number of parameters.

Weibull model Dose-response model of the form $P(d) = 1 - \exp(-bd^{m})$, where *P*(*d*) is the probability of response due to a continuous dose rate *d*; and b and m are constants. The model is useful for extrapolating from high- to low-dose exposures, e.g., from animals to human.

Weighted average A value determined by assigning weights to individual measurements. Each value is assigned a nonnegative coefficient (weight); the sum of the products of each value by its weight divided by the sum of the weights is the weighted average.

Weighted kappa A version of the kappa coefficient that allows disagreements between raters to be differentially weighted to allow differences in how serious such disagreements are judged to be.

Weighted least squares A method of estimation in which estimates arise from minimizing a weighted sum of squares of the differences between the response variable and its predicted value in terms of the model of interest. Often used when the variance of the response variable is thought to change over the range of values of the explanatory variable(s), in which case the weights are generally taken as the reciprocals of the variance.

Weight variation tests Tests designed to ensure that manufacturers control the variation in the weights of the tablet forms of the drugs that they produce.

Wilcoxon's rank sum test Another name for the *Mann-Whitney test.*

Wilcoxon's signed rank test A distribution-free method for testing the difference between two populations by using matched samples. The test is based on the absolute differences of the pairs of observations in the two samples ranked according to size, with each rank being given the sign of the original difference.

Wilk's multivariate outlier test A test for detecting outliers in multivariate data that assumes that the data arise from a multivariate normal distribution.

William's test A test used to answer questions about the toxicities of substances and at what dose level any toxicity occurs. The test assumes that the mean response of the variate is a monotonic function of dose.

Yates' correction An adjustment proposed by Yates in the chi-square calculation for a two-by-two contingency table that subtracts 0.5 from the positive discrepancies (observed – expected) and adding 0.5 to the negative discrepancies before these values are squared in the calculation of the usual chi-square statistic. This brings the distribution based on the discontinuous frequencies closer to the continuous chi-square distribution from which the published tables for testing chi-square values are derived.

Zelen's single-consent design A modified double-blind randomized controlled trial design for the formation of treatment groups in a clinical trial. The essential feature is randomization before informed consent procedures, which is claimed to be needed only for the group allocated to receive the experimental regimen.

z test A test for assessing hypotheses about population means when their variances are known. If the null hypothesis is true, z has a standard normal distribution.

SOURCES

Dorland's Illustrated Medical Dictionary, 28th edition. 1994. Philadelphia: W. B. Saunders.

Eddy, D. M., V. Hasselblad, and R. Shacther. 1992. *Meta-Analysis by the Confidence Profile Method.* San Diego: Academic Press.

Everitt, B. S. 1995. *The Cambridge Dictionary of Statistics in the Medical Sciences.* Cambridge, United Kingdom: Cambridge University Press.

Hirsch, R. P., and R. Riegelman. 1996. *Statistical Operations. Analysis of Health Research Data.* Cambridge, MA: Blackwell Science.

Last, J. M., ed. 1995. *A Dictionary of Epidemiology.* Oxford: Oxford University Press.

Appendix C
Selected Bibliography on Small Clinical Trials

This bibliography is a selection of published references dealing with analytical approaches and statistical methods applicable to clinical trials, particularly small clinical trials. The citations span the field broadly and are the result of searches of the Medline database and suggestions from the committee and from the experts in the field who made presentations at the committee's invitational workshop. The references are organized into specific categories to aid the reader. Although comprehensive, the list is selective, and the committee believes that it is an up-to-date bibliography that will assist researchers in learning more about design and analytical methods applicable to small clinical trials.

GENERAL

Bohning, D. 1999. *Computer-Assisted Analysis of Mixtures and Applications: Meta-Analysis, Disease Mapping, and Others.* Boca Raton, FL: Chapman & Hall/CRC.

Cai, J., H. Zhou, and C. E. Davis. 1997. Estimating the mean hazard ratio parameters for clustered survival data with random clusters. *Statistics in Medicine* 16:2009–2020.

D'Agostino, R. B., and H. Kwan. 1995. *Measuring effectiveness. What to expect without a randomized control group.* Medical Care 33(Suppl. 4):AS95–AS105.

Davis, C. E. 1997. Secondary endpoints can be validly analyzed, even if the primary endpoint does not provide clear statistical significance. *Controlled Clinical Trials* 18:557–560.

Davis, C. E., S. Hunsberger, D. M. Murray, R. R. Fabsitz, J. H. Himes, L. K. Stephenson, B. Caballero, and B. Skipper. 1999. Design and statistical analysis for the Pathways study. *American Journal of Clinical Nutrition* 69(Suppl. 4):S760–S763.

Dieterich, M., S. N. Goodman, R. R. Rojas-Corona, A. B. Emralino, J, D, Jimenez, and M. E. Sherman. 1994. Multivariate analysis of prognostic features in malignant pleural effusions from breast cancer patients. *Acta Cytologica* 38:945–952.

Everitt, B. S. 1994. *Statistical Methods in Medical Investigations.* New York: Halsted Press.

Everitt, B. S. 1995. *The Cambridge Dictionary of Statistics in the Medical Sciences.* New York: Cambridge University Press.

Gehan, E. A. 1965. A generalized two-sample Wilcoxon test for doubly censored data. *Biometrika* 52:650–653.

Gehan, E. A., and N. A. Lemak. 1994. *Statistics in Medical Research: Developments in Clinical Trials.* New York: Plenum Medical Book Co.

Gibbons, J. D., I. Olkin, and M. Sobel. 1999. *Selecting and Ordering Populations: A New Statistical Methodology.* Philadelphia: SIAM.

Gilbert, P. B., S. G. Self, and M. A. Ashby. 1998. Statistical methods for assessing differential vaccine protection against human immunodeficiency virus types. *Biometrics* 54:799–814.

Goodman, S. N. 1992. A comment on replication, *p*-values and evidence. *Statistics in Medicine* 11:875–879.

Goodman, S. N. 1993. *P* values, hypothesis tests, and likelihood: implications for epidemiology of a neglected historical debate. *American Journal of Epidemiology* 137:485–496; (Discussion, 137:497–501).

Goodman, S. N. 1994. Confidence limits vs power, calculations. *Epidemiology* 5:266–268. (Discussion, 5:268–269.

Goodman, S. N. 1999. Toward evidence-based medical statistics. 1. The *P* value fallacy. *Annals of Internal Medicine* 130:995–1004.

Goodman, S. N. 1999. Toward evidence-based medical statistics. 2. The Bayes factor. *Annals of Internal Medicine* 130:1005–1013.

Goodman, S. N., and J. A. Berlin. 1994. The use of predicted confidence intervals when planning experiments and the misuse of power when interpreting results. *Annals of Internal Medicine* 121:200–206.

Goodman, S. N., D. G. Altman, and S. L. George. 1998. Statistical reviewing policies of medical journals: caveat lector? *Journal of General Internal Medicine* 13:753–756.

Halloran, M. E., and D. Berry, eds. 2000. *Statistical Models in Epidemiology, the Environment, and Clinical Trials. The Ima Volumes in Mathematics and Its Applications*, Vol. 116. New York: Springer-Verlag.

Hoppensteadt, F. C., and C. S. Peskin. 1992. *Mathematics in Medicine and the Life Sciences.* New York: Springer-Verlag.

Ildstad, S. T., D. J. Tollerud, M. E. Bigelow, and J. P. Remensnyder. 1989. A multivariate analysis of determinants of survival for patients with squamous cell carcinoma of the head and neck. *Annals of Surgery* 209:237–41.

Jennison, C., and B. W. Turnbull. 1983. Confidence intervals for a binomial parameter following a multistage test with application to MIL-STD 105D and medical trials. *Technometrics* 25:49–58.

Khoury, M. J., T. H. Beaty, and B. H. Cohen. 1993. *Fundamentals of Genetic*

Epidemiology. Monographs in Epidemiology and Biostatistics, Vol. 22. New York: Oxford University Press.

Knapp, R. G., and M. C. Miller. 1992. *Clinical Epidemiology and Biostatistics (The National Medical Series for Independent Study).* Baltimore: Williams & Wilkins.

Kramer, M. S. 1988. *Clinical Epidemiology and Biostatistics: A Primer for Clinical Investigators and Decision-Makers.* New York: Springer-Verlag.

Last, J. ed. 1995. *A Dictionary of Epidemilogy* (Edited for the International Epidemiological Association). New York: Oxford University Press.

Lazaridis, E., and R. Gonin. 1997. Continuously monitored stopping boundary methodologies: The issues of sensitivity, association and trial suspension. *Statistics in Medicine* 16:1925–1941.

Levin, B. 1986. Empirical Bayes' estimation in heterogeneous matched binary samples with systematic aging effects. In: *Adaptive Statistical Procedure and Related Topics.* J. van Ryzin, ed. *Institute of Mathematics and Statistics Lecture Notes—Monograph Series* 8:179–194.

Levin, B. 1987. Conditional likelihood analysis in stratum-matched retrospective studies with polytomous disease states. *Communications in Statistics* 16:699–718.

Levin, B. 1990. The saddlepoint correction in conditional logistic likelihood analysis. *Biometrika* 77:275–285.

Levin, B., and F. Kong. 1990. Barlett's bias correction to the profile score function is a saddlepoint correction. *Biometrika* 77:219–221.

Levin, B., and H. Robbins. 1981. Selecting the highest probability in binomial or multinomial trials. *Proceedings of the National Academy of Sciences* USA 78:4663–4666.

Liang, K. Y., S. G. Self, K. J. Bandeen-Roche, and S. L. Zeger. 1995. Some recent developments for regression analysis of multivariate failure time data. *Lifetime Data Analysis* 1:403–415.

McPherson, G. 1990. Statistical analysis: the statistician's view. Pp. 154–180 In: *Statistics in Scientific Investigation. Its Basis, Application, and Interpretation.* New York: Springer-Verlag.

McPherson, G. 1990. Studying association and correlation. Pp. 475–508 In: *Statistics in Scientific Investigation. Its Basis, Application, and Interpretation.* New York: Springer-Verlag.

Meinert, C. L., 1986. *Clinical Trials: Design, Conduct, and Analysis.* New York: Oxford University Press.

Murray, D. M. 1998. *Design and Analysis of Group-Randomized Trials. Monographs in Epidemiology and Biostatistics*, Vol. 29. New York: Oxford University Press.

O'Quigley, J., and L. Z. Shen. 1996. Continual reassessment method: a likelihood approach. *Biometrics* 52:673–684.

Petitti, D. B. 1994. *Meta-Analysis, Decision Analysis, and Cost-Effectiveness Analysis: Methods for Quantitative Synthesis in Medicine.* New York: Oxford University Press.

Pham, B., A. Cranney, M. Boers, A. C. Verhoeven, G. Wells, and P. Tugwell. 1999. Validity of area-under-the-curve analysis to summarize effect in rheumatoid arthritis clinical trials. *Journal of Rheumatology* 26:712–716.

Racine-Poon, A., and J. Wakefield. 1998. Statistical methods for population pharmacokinetic modelling. *Statistical Methods in Medical Research* 7:63–84.

Sevin, S. 1996. *Statistical Analysis of Epidemiologic Data. Monographs in Epidemiology and Biostatistics*, Vol. 25. New York: Oxford University Press.
Sevin, S. 1998. *Modern Applied Biostatistical Methods: Using S-Plus. Monographs in Epidemiology and Biostatistics*, Vol. 28. New York: Oxford University Press.
Stroup, D. F. 1999. Symposium on Statistical Bases for Public Health Decision Making: From Exploration to Modelling. Closing remarks. *Statistics in Medicine* 18:3373–3375.
Tersmette, A. C., S. N. Goodman, G. J. Offerhaus, K. W. Tersmette, F. M. Giardcllo, J. P. Vandenbroucke, and G. N. Tytgat. 1991. Multivariate analysis of the risk of stomach cancer after ulcer surgery in an Amsterdam cohort of postgasterectomy patients. *American Journal of Epidemiology* 134:14–21.
Weinstein, G. S., and B. Levin. 1989. The effect of cross-over on the statistical power of randomized studies. *Annals of Thoracic Surgery* 48:490–495.
Weiss, N. S. 1996. *Clinical Epidemiology: The Study of the Outcome of Illness. Monographs in Epidemiology and Biostatistics*, Vol. 27. New York: Oxford University Press.
Zeger, S. L. 1991. Statistical reasoning in epidemiology. *American Journal of Epidemiology* 134:1062–1066.
Zeger, S. L., and S. D. Harlow. 1987. Mathematical models from laws of growth to tools for biologic analysis: fifty years of "Growth". *Growth* 51:1–21.
Zeger, S. L. and J. Katz. 1994. Estimation of design effects in cluster surveys. *Annals of Epidemiology* 4:295–301.
Zeger, S. L., and K.Y. Liang. 1993. Regression analysis for correlated data. *Annual Review of Public Health* 14:43–68.
Zeger, S. L., and A. Sommer. 1991. On estimating efficacy from clinical trials. *Statistics in Medicine* 10:45–52.
Zeger, S. L., L. C. See, and P. J. Diggle. 1989. Statistical methods for monitoring the AIDS epidemic. *Statistics in Medicine* 8:3–21.
Zeger, S. L., C. B. Hall, and K. J. Bandeen-Roche. 1996. Adjusted variable plots for Cox's proportional hazards regression model. *Lifetime Data Analysis* 2:73–90.
Zeger, S. L., D. Thomas, F. Dominici, J. M. Samet, J. Schwartz, D. Dockery, and A. Cohen. 2000. Exposure measurement error in time-series studies of air pollution: concepts and consequences. *Environmental Health Perspective* 108:419–426.

SAMPLE SIZE

Brunier, H. C., and J. Whitehead. 1994. Sample sizes for phase II clinical trials derived from Bayesian decision theory. *Statistics in Medicine* 13:2493–2502.
Flournoy, N., and I. Olkin. 1995. Do small trials square with large ones? *The Lancet* 345:741–742.
Gehan, E. A. 1961. The determination of the number of patients required in a preliminary and a follow-up trial of a new chemotherapeutic agent. *Journal of Chronic Disease* 13:346–353.
Gould, A. L. 1995. Planning and revising the sample size for a trial. *Statistics in Medicine* 14:1039–1051.
Hanfelt, J. J., R. S. Slack, and E. A. Gehan. 1999. A modification of Simon's optimal design for phase II trials when the criterion is median sample size. *Controlled Clinical Trials* 20:555–566.

Kim, K., and D. L. DeMets. 1992. Sample size determination for group sequential clinical trials with immediate response. *Statistics in Medicine* 11:1391–1399.

McMahon, R. P., M. Proschan, N. L. Geller, P. H. Stone, and G. Sopko. 1994. Sample size calculation for clinical trials in which entry criteria and outcomes are counts of events. *Statistics in Medicine* 13:859–870.

Mehta, C. R., N. R. Patel, and P. Senchaudhuri. 1998. Exact power and sample-size computations for the Cochran-Armitage trend test. *Biometrics* 54:1615–1621.

Rochon, J. 1998. Application of GEE procedures for sample size calculations in repeated measures experiments. *Statistics in Medicine* 17:1643–1658.

Simon, R. M., and R. W. Makuch. 1982. Sample size requirements for comparing time-to-failure among *k* treatment groups. *Journal of Chronic Disease* 35:861–867.

Stallard, N. 1998. Sample size determination for phase II clinical trials based on Bayesian decision theory. *Biometrics* 54:279–294.

Wels, G., A. Cranney, B. Shea, and P. Tugwell. 1997. Responsiveness of endpoints in osteoporosis clinical trials. *Journal of Rheumatology* 24:1230–1233.

Whitehead, J. 1985. Designing phase II studies in the context of a programme of clinical research. *Biometrics* 41:373–383.

Whitehead, J. 1986. Sample sizes for phase II and phase III clinical trials: an integrated approach. *Statistics in Medicine* 5(5):459-464.

Whitehead, J. 1996. Sample sizes calculations for ordered categorical data. *Statistics in Medicine* 15:1065–1066.

Whitehead, J., K. Bolland, and M.R. Sooriyarachchi. 1998. Sample size review in a head injury trial with ordered categorical responses. *Statistics in Medicine* 17:2835–2847.

Wolfe, R., and J. B. Carlin. 1999. Sample-size calculation for log-transformed outcome measure. *Controlled Clinical Trials* 20:547–554.

CLINICAL TRIALS

Begg, C., M. Cho, S. Eastwood, R. Horton, D. Moher, I. Olkin, R. Pitkin, D. Rennie, K. F. Schulz, D. Simel, and D. F. Stroup. 1996. Improving the quality of reporting of randomized controlled trials. The CONSORT statement. *Journal of the American Medical Association* 276:637–639.

Benson, K., and A. J. Hartz. 2000. A comparison of observational studies and randomized, controlled trials. *New England Journal of Medicine* 342:1878–1886.

Black, H. R., W. J. Elliott, J. D. Neaton, G. Grandits, P. Grambsch, R. H. Grimm, Jr., L. Hansson, Y. Lacouciere, J. Muller, P. Sleight, M. A. Weber, W. B. White, G. Williams, J. Wittes, A. Zanchetti, and T. D. Fakouhi. 1998. Rationale and design for the Controlled Onset Verapamil Investigation of Cardiovascular Endpoints (CONVINCE) trial. *Controlled Clinical Trials* 19:370–390.

Bombardier, C., and P. Tugwell. 1985. Controversies in the analysis of long term clinical trials of slow acting drugs. *Journal of Rheumatology* 12:403–405.

Buyse, M., S. L. George, S. Evans, N. L. Geller, J. Ranstam, B. Scherrer, E. Lesaffre, G. Murray, L. Edler, J. Hutton, T. Colton, P. Lachenbruch, and B. L. Verma. 1999. The role of biostatistics in the prevention, detection and treatment of fraud in clinical trials. *Statistics in Medicine* 18:3435–3451.

Concato, J., N. Shah, and R. I. Horwitz. 2000. Randomized, controlled trials, observational studies, and the hierarchy of research designs. *New England Journal of Medicine* 342:1887–1892.

Cranney, A., P. Tugwell, S. Cummings, P. Sambrook, J. Adachi, A. J. Silman, W. J. Gillespie, D. T. Felson, B. Shea, and G. Wells. 1997. Osteoporosis clinical trials endpoints: candidate variables and clinimetric properties. *Journal of Rheumatology* 24:1222–1229.

DeMets, D. L. 1987. Practical aspects in data monitoring: a brief overview. *Statistics in Medicine* 6:753–760.

DeMets, D. L. 1990. Methodological issues in AIDS clinical trials. Data monitoring and sequential analysis—an academic perspective. *Journal of Acquired Immune Deficiency Syndrome* 3(Suppl. 2):S124–S133.

DeMets, D. L. 1997. Distinction between fraud, bias, errors, misunderstanding, and incompetence. *Controlled Clinical Trials* 18:637–650. (Discussion, 661–666.)

DeMets, D. L., and M. Halperin. 1982. Early stopping in the two-sample problem for bounded random variables. *Controlled Clinical Trials* 3:1–11.

DeMets, D. L., and C. L. Meinert. 1991. Data integrity. *Controlled Clinical Trials* 12:727–730.

DeMets, D. L., S. J. Pocock, and D. G. Julian. 1999. The agonizing negative trend in monitoring clinical trials. *The Lancet* 354:1983–1988.

Elliott, T. E., R. P. Dinapoli, J. R. O'Fallon, J. E. Krook, J. D. Earle, R. F. Morton, R. Levitt, L. K. Tschetter, B. W. Scheithauer, D. M. Pfeifle, D. I. Twito, and R. A. Nelimark. 1997. Randomized trial of radiation therapy (RT) plus dibromodulcitol (DBD) versus RT plus BCNU in high grade astrocytoma. *Journal of Neurooncology* 33:239–250.

Estey, E. 1997. Prognostic factors in clinical cancer trials. *Clinical Cancer Research* 3:2591–2593.

Fine, J., J. Duff, R. Chen, W. Hutchison, A. M. Lozano, and A. E. Lang. 2000. Long-term follow-up of unilateral pallidotomy in advanced Parkinson's disease. *New England Journal of Medicine* 342:1708–1714.

Finkelstein, M. O., B. Levin, and H. Robbins. 1996. Clinical and prophylactic trials with assured new treatment for those at greater risk. I. A design proposal. *American Journal of Public Health* 86:691–695.

Finkelstein, M. O., B. Levin, and H. Robbins. 1996. Clinical and prophylactic trials with assured new treatment for those at greater risk: II. Examples. *American Journal of Public Health* 86:696–705.

Fleming, T. R. 1990. Evaluation of active control trials in AIDS. *Journal of Acquired Immune Deficiency Syndrome* 3(Suppl. 2):S82–S87.

Fleming, T. R. 1994. Surrogate markers in AIDS and cancer trials. *Statistics in Medicine* 13:1423–1435. (Discussion 13:1437–1440).

Fleming, T. R. 1999. Issues in the design of clinical trials: insights from the trastuzumab (Herceptin) experience. *Seminar in Oncology* 26(4 Suppl. 12):102–107.

Fleming, T. R. 2000. Design and interpretation of equivalence trials. *American Heart Journal* 139:171–176.

Fleming, T. R., V. DeGruttola, and D. L. DeMets. 1998. Surrogate endpoints. In: *AIDS Clinical Review 1997/1998*. P. A. Volberding and M. A. Jacobson, eds. New York: Marcel Dekker.

Fleming, T. R., and D. L. DeMets. 1993. Monitoring of clinical trials: issues and recommendations. *Controlled Clinical Trials* 14:183–197.

Fleming, T. R., and D. L. DeMets. 1996. Surrogate endpoints in clinical trials: are we being misled? *Annals of Internal Medicine* 125:605–613.

Fleming, T. R., and S. J. Green. 1988. Guidelines for the reporting of clinical trials. *Seminars in Oncology* 15:455–461.

Fleming, T. R., S. J. Green, and D. P. Harrington. 1984. Considerations for monitoring and evaluating treatment effects in clinical trials. *Controlled Clinical Trials* 5:55–66.

Fleming, T. R., R. L. Prentice, M. S. Pepe, and D. Glidden. 1994. Surrogate and auxiliary endpoints in clinical trials, with potential applications in cancer and AIDS research. *Statistics in Medicine* 13:955–968.

Fleming, T. R., J. D. Neaton, A. Goldman, D. L. DeMets, C. Launer, J. Korvick, and D. Abrams. 1995. Insights from monitoring the CPCRA didanosine/xalcitabine trial. *Journal of Acquired Immune Deficiency Syndrome.* 10 (Suppl. 2):S9–S18.

Fleming, T. R., and L. F. Watelet. 1989. Approaches to monitoring clinical trials. *Journal of the National Cancer Institute* 81:188–193.

Foote, L. R., C. L. Loprinzi, A. R. Frank, J. R. O'Fallon, S. Gulavita, H. H. Tewfik, M. A. Ryan, J. M. Earle, and P. Novotny. 1994. Randomized trial of a chlorhexidine mouthwash for alleviation of radiation-induced mucositis. *Journal of Clinical Oncology* 12:2630–2633.

Gazarian, M., P. Tugwell, M. Boers, C. Bombardier, P. Brooks, R. Day, V. Strand, and G. Wells. 1999. Patient based methods for assessing adverse events in clinical trials in rheumatology. Progress Report for OMERACT Drug Toxicity Working Party Outcome Measures in Rheumatology. *Journal of Rheumatology* 26:207–209.

Gehan, E. A. 1978. Comparative clinical trials with historical controls: a statistician's view. *Biomedicine* 28:13–19.

Gehan, E. A. 1982. Design of controlled clinical trials: use of historical controls. *Cancer Treatment Reports* 66:1089–1093.

Gehan, E. A. 1986. Update on planning of Phase II clinical trials. *Drugs Under Experimental and Clinical Research* 12:43–50.

Gehan, E. A. 1988. Methodological issues in cancer clinical trials: the comparison of therapies. *Biomedicine and Pharmacotherapy* 42:161–165.

Gehan, E. A. 1997. The scientific basis of clinical trials: statistical aspects. *Clinical Cancer Research* 3(12 Pt 2):2587–2590.

Gehan, E. A., and E. J. Freireich. 1981. Cancer clinical trials. A rational basis for use of historical controls. *Seminars in Oncology* 8:430–436.

Gehan, E. A., and M. A. Schneiderman. 1990. Historical and methodological developments in clinical trials at the National Cancer Institute. *Statistics in Medicine* 9:871–880. (Discussion, 903–906.)

Gehan, E. A., L. G. Ensign, D. S. Kamen, and P. F. Thall. 1994. An optimal three-stage design for phase II clinical trials. *Statistics in Medicine* 13:1727–1736.

Goldberg, R. M., C. L. Loprinzi, J. A. Mailliard, J. R. O'Fallon, J. E. Krook, C. Ghosh, R. D. Hestorff, S. F. Chong, N. F. Reuter, and T. G. Shanahan. 1995. Pentoxifylline for treatment of cancer anorexia and cachexia? A randomized, double-blind, placebo-controlled trial. *Journal of Clinical Oncology* 13:2856–2859.

Green, L. A., F. S. Rhame, R. W. Price, D. C. Perlman, L. G. Capps, J. H. Sampson, L. R. Deyton, S. M. Schnittman, E. J. Fisher, G. E. Bartsch, E. A. Krum, and J. D. Neaton.

1998. Experience with a cross-study endpoint review committee for AIDS clinical trials. *AIDS* 12:1983–1990.
Heitjan, D. F. 1999. Ignorability and bias in clinical trials. *Statistics in Medicine* 18:2421–2434.
Herson, J. 1979. Predictive probability early termination plans for phase II clinical trials. *Biometrics* 35:775–783.
Herson, J., and S. K. Carter. 1986. Calibrated phase II clinical trials in oncology. *Statistics in Medicine* 5:441–447.
Institute of Medicine. 1990. *Modern Methods of Clinical Investigation.* Washington, DC: National Academy Press.
Kessler, D. A., J. P. Siegel, P. D. Noguchi, K. C. Zoon, K. L. Feiden, and J. Woodcock. 1993. Regulation of somatic-cell therapy and gene therapy by the Food and Drug Administration. *New England Journal of Medicine* 329:1169–1173.
Keyserling, T. C., A. S. Ammerman, C. E. Davis, M. C. Mok, J. Garrett, and R. Simpson, Jr. 1997. A randomized controlled trial of a physician-directed treatment program for low-income patients with high blood cholesterol: the Southeast Cholesterol Project. *Archives of Family Medicine* 6:135–145.
Knatterud, G. L., F. W. Rockhold, S. L. George, F. B. Barton, C. E. Davis, W. R. Fairweather, T. Honohan, R. Mowery, and R. O'Neill. 1998. Guidelines for quality assurance in multicenter trials: a position paper. *Controlled Clinical Trials* 19:477–493.
Lazaridis, E. N. and R. Gonin. 1997. Continuously monitored stopping boundary methodologies: the issues of sensitivity, association and trial suspension. *Statistics in Medicine* 16:1925–1941.
Lin, D. Y., T. R. Fleming, and V. De Grutolla. 1997. Estimating the proportion of treatment effect explained by a surrogate marker. *Statistics in Medicine* 16:1515–1527.
Loprinzi, C. L., L. M. Athman, C. G. Kardinal, J. R. O'Fallon, J. A. See, B. K. Bruce, A. M. Dose, A. W. Miser, P. S. Kern, L. K. Tschetter, and S. Rayson. 1996. Randomized trial of dietician counseling to try to prevent weight gain associated with breast cancer adjuvant chemotherapy. *Oncology* 53:228–232.
Loprinzi, C. L., S. A. Kuross, J. T. O'Fallon, D. H. Gesme, Jr., J. B. Gerstner, R. M. Rospond, C. D. Cobau, and R. M. Goldberg. 1994. Randomized placebo-controlled trial evaluation of hydrazine sulfate in patients with colorectal cancer. *Journal of Clinical Oncology* 12:1121–1125.
Mahe, C., and S. Chevret. 1999. Estimation of the treatment effect in a clinical trial when recurrent events define the endpoint. *Statistics in Medicine* 18:1821–1829.
Martenson, J. A., Jr., G. Hyland, C. G. Moertel, J. A. Mailliard, J. R. O'Fallon, R. T. Collins, R. F. Morton, H. H. Tewfik, R. L. Moore,A. R. Frank, R. E. Urias, and R. L. Deming. 1996. Olsalazine is contraindicated during pelvic radiation therapy: results of a double-blind, randomized clinical trial. *International Journal of Radiation Oncology, Biology and Physics* 35:299–303.
Matthews, J. N. S. 1995. Small clinical trials: are they all bad? *Statistics in Medicine* 14:115-126.
May, G. S., D. L. DeMets, L. M. Friedman, C. Furberg, and E. Passamani. 1981. The randomized clinical trial: bias in analysis. *Circulation* 64:669–673.
Moher, D., A. R. Jadad, and P. Tugwell. 1996. Assessing the quality of randomized

controlled trials. Current issues and future directions. *International Journal of Technology Assessment and Health Care* 12:195–208.

Morgan, J. M., D. M. Capuzzi, J. R. Guyton, R. M. Centor, R. Goldberg, D. C. Robbins, D. DiPette, S. Jenkins, and S. Marcovina. 1996. Treatment effect of Niaspan, a controlled-release niacin, in patients with hypercholesterolemia: a placebo-controlled trial. *Journal of Cardiovascular Pharmacology and Therapeutics* 1:195–202.

Mosteller, F. 1996. The promise of risk-based allocation trials in assessing new treatments. *American Journal of Public Health* 86:622–623.

Neaton, J. D., and G. E. Bartsch. 1992. Impact of measurement error and temporal variability on the estimation of event probabilities for risk factor intervention trials. *Statistics in Medicine* 11:1719–1729.

Neaton, J. D., A. G. Duchene, K. H. Svendsen, and D. Wentworth. 1990. An examination of the efficiency of some quality assurance methods commonly employed in clinical trials. *Statistics in Medicine* 9:115–123. (Discussion, 124.)

Neaton, J. D., G. E. Bartsch, S. K. Broste, J. D. Cohen, and N. M. Simon. 1991. A case of data alteration in the Multiple Risk Factor Intervention Trial (MRFIT). *Controlled Clinical Trials* 12:731–740.

Neaton, J. D., D. N. Wentworth, F. Rhame, C. Hogan, D. I. Abrams, and L. Deyton. 1994. Considerations in choice of a clinical endpoint for AIDS clinical trials. *Statistics in Medicine* 13:2107–2125.

Pocock, S. J., and D. R. Elbourne. 2000. Randomized trials or observational tribulations? *New England Journal of Medicine* 342:1907–1909.

Pocock, S. J., N. L. Geller, and A. A. Tsiatis. 1987. The analysis of multiple endpoints in clinical trials. *Biometrics* 43:487–498.

Schaper, C., T. R. Fleming, S. G. Self, and W. N. Rida. 1995. Statistical issues in the design of HIV vaccine trials. *Annual Review of Public Health* 16:1–22.

Shapiro, A. M. J., J. R. T. Lakey, E. A. Ryan, G. S. Korbutt, E. Toth, G. L. Warnock, N. M. Kneteman, and R. V. Rajotte. 2000. Islet transplantation in seven patients with type I diabetes mellitus using a glucocorticoid-free immunosuppressive regimen. *New England Journal of Medicine* 343:230–238

Sharples, K., T. R. Fleming, S. MacMahon, A. Moore, I. Reid, and B. Scoggins. 1998. Monitoring clinical trials. *New Zealand Medical Journal* 111:322–325.

Shen, Y., and T. R. Fleming. 1999. Assessing effects on long-term survival after early termination of randomized trials. *Lifetime Data Analysis* 5:55–66.

Siegel, J. P. 2000. Equivalence and noninferiority trials. *American Heart Journal* 139:S166–S170.

Sloan, J. A., C. L. Loprinzi, S. A. Kuross, A. W. Miser, J. R. O'Fallon, M. R. Mahoney, I. M. Heid, M. E. Bretscher, and N. L. Vaught. 1998. Randomized comparison of four tools measuring overall quality of life in patients with advanced cancer. *Journal of Clinical Oncology* 16:3662–3673.

Sposto, R., and D. O. Stram. 1999. A strategic view of randomized trial design in low-incidence pediatric cancer. *Statistics in Medicine* 18:1183–1197.

Thall, P. F., and R. M. Simon. 1995. Recent developments in the design of phase II clinical trials. In: *Recent Advances in Clinical Trial Design and Analysis*. P. F. Thall, ed. Boston: Kluwer.

Thall, P. F., R. M. Simon, and E. H. Estey. 1996. New statistical strategy for monitoring safety and efficacy in single-arm clinical trials. *Journal of Clinical Oncology* 14:296–303.

Tsai, J. F., L.M. Li, and J. K. Chen. 2000. Reconstruction of damaged cornea by transplantation of autologous limbal epithelial cells. *New England Journal of Medicine* 343:86–93.

Vico, L., P. Collet, A. Guignandon, M. H. Lafage-Proust, T. Thomas, M. Rehailia, and C. Alexandre. 2000. Effects of long-term microgravity exposure on cancellous and cortical weight-bearing bones of cosmonauts. *The Lancet* 355:1607–1611.

Whitehead, J. 1993. The case for frequentism in clinical trials. *Statistics in Medicine* 12:1405–1413. (Discussion, 12:1415–1419.)

Whitehead, J. 1999. Stopping a clinical trial properly. *The Lancet* 353:2164. (Comments, 353:943–944.)

Whitehead, J. 2000. Monitoring and evaluating clinical trials data. *Intensive Care Medicine* 26 (Suppl. 1):S84–S88.

Whitehead, J., and M. Mittlbock. 1998. The interpretation of clinical trials of immediate versus delayed therapy. *Lifetime Data Analysis* 4:253–263.

Whitehead, J., D. G. Altman, M.K. Parmar, S.P. Stenning, P.M. Fayers, and D. Machin. 1995. Randomised consent designs in cancer clinical trials. *European Journal of Cancer* 31A:1934–1944.

PHASE I CLINICAL TRIALS

Ahn, C. 1998. An evaluation of phase I cancer clinical trial designs. *Statistics in Medicine* 17:1537–1549.

Babb, J., A. Rogatko, and S. Zacks. 1998. Cancer phase I clinical trials: efficient dose escalation with overdose control. *Statistics in Medicine* 17:1103–1120.

Berlin, J., J. A. Stewart, B. Storer, K. D. Tusch, R. Z. Arzoomanian, D. Alberti, C. Feierabend, K. Simon, and G. Wilding. 1998. Phase I clinical and pharmacokinetic trial of penclomedine using a novel, two-stage trial design for patients with advanced malignancy. *Journal of Clinical Oncology* 16:1142–1149.

Durham, S. D., N. Flournoy, and W. F. Rosenberger. 1997. A random walk rule for phase I clinical trials. *Bioemetrics* 53:745–760.

Geller, N. L. 1984. Design of phase I and II clinical trials in cancer: a statistician's view. *Cancer Investigation* 2:483–491.

Goodman, S. N., M. L. Zahurak, and S. Piantadosi. 1995. Some practical improvements in the continual reassessment method for phase I studies. *Statistics in Medicine* 14:1149–1161.

Gordon, N. H., and J. K. Willson. 1992. Using toxicity grades in the design and analysis of cancer phase I clinical trials. *Statistics in Medicine* 11:2063–2075.

Hageboutros, A., A. Rogatko, E. M. Newman, C. McAleer, J. Brennan, F. P. LaCreta, G. R. Hudes, R. F. Ozols, and P. J. O'Dwyer. 1995. Phase I study of phosphonacetyl-l-aspartate, 5-fluorouracil, and leucovorin patients with advanced cancer. *Cancer Chemotherapy and Pharmacology* 35:205–212.

Heyd, J. M., and B. P. Carlin. 1999. Adaptive design improvements in the continual reassessment method for phase I studies. *Statistics in Medicine* 18:1307–1321.

Korn, E. L., D. Midthune, T. T. Chen, L. V. Rubinstein, M. C. Christian, and R. M. Simon. 1994. A comparison of two phase I trial designs. *Statistics in Medicine* 13:1799–1806.

Kramar, A., A. Lebecq, and E. Candalh. 1999. Continual reassessment methods in phase I trials of the combination of the two drugs in oncology. *Statistics in Medicine* 18:1849–1864.

Lin, H. M., and M. D. Hughes. 1995. Use of historical marker data for assessing treatment effects in phase I/II trials when subject selection is determined by baseline marker level. *Biometrics* 51:1053–1063.

O'Dwyer, P. J., T. C. Hamilton, F. P. LaCreta, J. M. Gallo, D. Kilpatrick, T. Halbherr, J. Brennan, M. A. Bookman, J. Hoffman, R. C. Young, R. L. Comis, and R. F. Ozols. 1996. Phase I trial of buthionine sulfoximine in combination with melphalan in patients with cancer. *Journal of Clinical Oncology* 14:249–256.

O'Quigley, J. 1992. Estimating the probability of toxicity at the recommended dose following a phase I clinical trial in cancer. *Biometrics* 48:853–862.

O'Quigley, J., L. Z. Shen, and A. Gamst. 1999. Two-sample continual reassessment method. *Journal of Biopharmaceutical Statistics* 9:17–44.

O'Quigley, J., M. Pepe, and L. Fisher. 1990. Continual reassessment method: a practical design for phase I clinical trials in cancer. *Biometrics* 46:33–48.

Savarese, D. M., A. M. Denicoff, S. L. Berg, M. Hillig, S. P. Baker, J. A. O'Shauhnessy, C. Chow, G. A. Otterson, F. M. Balis, and D. G. Poplack. 1993. Phase I study of high-dose piroxantrone with granulocyte colony-stimulating factor. *Journal of Clinical Oncology* 11:1795–1803.

Simon, R., B. Freidlin, L. Rubinstein, S. G. Arbuck, J. Collins, and M. C. Christian. 1997. Accelerated titration designs for phase I clinical trials in oncology. *Journal of the National Cancer Institute* 89:1138–1147.

Smith, T. L., J. J. Lee, H. M. Kantarjian, S. S. Legha, and M. N. Raber. 1996. Design and results of phase I cancer clinical trials: three-year experience at M. D. Anderson Cancer Center. *Journal of Clinical Oncology* 14:287–295.

Storer, B. E. 1993. Small sample confidence sets for the MTD in phase I clinical trial. *Biometrics* 49:1117–1125.

Thall, P. F., and K. T. Russell. 1998. A strategy for dose-finding and safety monitoring based on efficacy and adverse outcomes in phase I/II clinical trials. *Biometrics* 54:251–264.

Thall, P. F., E. H. Estey, and H. G. Sung. 1999. A new statistical method for dose-finding based on efficacy and toxicity in early phase clinical trials. *Investigational New Drugs* 17:155–167.

Thall, P. F., J. J. Lee, C. H. Cheng, and E. H. Estey. 1999. Accrual strategies for phase I trials with delayed patient outcome. *Statistics in Medicine* 18:1155–1169.

PHASE III CLINICAL TRIALS

Bellamy, N., J. Kirwan, M. Boers, P. Brooks, V. Strand, P. Tugwell, R. Altman, K. Brandt, M. Dougados, and M. Lequesne. 1997. Recommendations for a core set of outcome measures for future phase III clinical trials in knee, hip, and hand osteoarthritis. Consensus development at OMERACT III. *Journal of Rheumatology* 24:799–802.

Bennett, C. L., R. Golub, T. M. Waters, M. S. Tallman, and J. M. Rowe. 1997. Economic analyses of phase III cooperative cancer group clinical trails: are they feasible? *Cancer Investigation* 15:227–236.

Desai, K. N., M. C. Boily, B. R. Masse, M. Alary, and R. M. Anderson. 1999. Simulation studies of phase III clinical trials to test the efficacy of a candidate HIV-1 vaccine. *Epidemiology and Infection* 123:65–88.

Dinapoli, R. P., L. D. Brown, R. M. Arusell, J. D. Earle, J. R. O'Fallon, J. C. Buckner, B. W. Scheithauer, J. E. Krook, L. K. Tschetter, and J. A. Maier. 1993. Phase III comparative evaluation of PCNU and carmustine combined with radiation therapy for high-grade glioma. *Journal of Clinical Oncology* 11:1316–1321.

Hand, J. W., D. Machin, C. C. Vernon, and J. B. Whaley. 1997. Analysis of thermal parameters obtained during phase III trials of hyperthermia as an adjunct to radiotherapy in the treatment of breast carcinoma. *International Journal of Hyperthermia* 13:343–364.

Morikawa, T., and M. Yoshida. 1995. A useful testing strategy in phase III trials: combined test of superiority and test of equivalence. *Journal of Biopharmaceutical Statistics* 5:297–306.

Palmer, C. R., and W. F. Rosenberger. 1999. Ethics and practice: alternative designs for phase III randomized clinical trials. *Controlled Clinical Trials* 20:172–186.

Sandler, A. B., J. Nemunaitis, C. Denham, J. von Pawel, Y. Cormier, U. Gartzemeier, K. Mattson, C. Manegold, M. C. Palmer, A. Gregor, B. Nguyen, C. Niyikiza, and L. H. Einhorn. 2000. Phase III trial of gemcitabine plus cisplatin versus cisplatin alone in patients with locally advanced or metastatic non-small-cell lung cancer. *Journal of Clinical Oncology* 18:122–130.

Williams, M. S., M. Burk, C. L. Loprinzi, M. Hill, P. J. Schomberg, K. Nearhood, J. R. O'Fallon, J. A. Laurie, T. G. Shanahan, R. L. Moore, R. E. Urias, R. R. Kuske, R. E. Engel, and W. D. Eggleston. 1996. Phase III double-blind evaluation of an aloe vera gel as a prophylactic agent for radiation-induced skin toxicity. *International Journal of Radiation Oncology, Biology and Physics* 36:345–349.

Yao, Q., and L. J. Wei. 1996. Play the winner for phase II/III clinical trials. *Statistics in Medicine* 15:2413–2423. (Discussion, 2455–2458.)

BAYESIAN APPROACH

Abrams, K., D. Ashby, and D. Errington. 1996. A Bayesian approach to Weibull survival models— application to a cancer clinical trial. *Lifetime Data Analysis* 2:159–174.

Berry, D. A. 1993. A case for Bayesianism in clinical trials. *Statistics in Medicine* 12:1377–1404.

Berry, D. A., and D. K. Stangl 1996. Bayesian methods in health-related research. In: *Bayesian Biostatistics*. D. A. Berry and D. K. Stangl, eds. New York: Marcel-Dekker.

Briggs, A. H. 1999. A Bayesian approach to stochastic cost-effectiveness analysis. *Health Economics* 8:257–261.

Brown, B. W., J. Herson, E. N. Atkinson, and M. E. Rozell. 1987. Projection from previous studies: a Bayesian and frequentist compromise. *Controlled Clinical Trials* 8:29–44.

Efron, B. 1986. Why isn't everyone a Bayesian? *American Statistician* 40:1–5.

Etzioni, R. D., and J. B. Kadane. 1995. Bayesian statistical methods in public health and medicine. *Annual Review of Public Health* 16:23–41.

Faraggi, D., and R. Simon. 1998. Bayesian variable selection method for censored survival data. *Biometrics* 54:1475–1485.

Fayers, P. M., D. Ashby, and M. K. Parmar. 1997. Tutorial in biostatistics Bayesian data monitoring in clinical trials. *Statistics in Medicine* 16:1413–1430.

Fisher, L. D. 1996. Comments on Bayesian and frequentist analysis and interpretation of clinical trials. *Controlled Clinical Trials* 17:423–434.

Freedman, L. S., and D. J. Spiegelhalter. 1989. Comparison of Bayesian with group sequential methods for monitoring clinical trials. *Controlled Clinical Trials* 10:357–367.

Greenhouse, J. B., and L. Wasserman. 1995. Robust Bayesian methods for monitoring clinical trials. *Statistics in Medicine* 14:1379–1391.

Gustafson, P. 1996. Robustness considerations in Bayesian analysis. *Statistical Methods in Medical Research*. 5:357–373.

Heitjan, D. F. 1997. Bayesian interim analysis of phase II cancer clinical trials. *Statistics in Medicine* 16:1791–1802.

Karim, M. R., and S. L. Zeger. 1992. Generalized linear models with random effects; salamander mating revisited. *Biometrics* 48:631–644.

Kleinman, K. P., and J. G. Ibrahim. 1998. A semiparametric Bayesian approach to the random effects model. *Biometrics* 54:921–938.

Kleinman, K. P., J. G. Ibrahim, and N. M. Laird. 1998. A Bayesian framework for intent-to-treat analysis with missing data. *Biometrics* 54:265–278.

Lehmann, H. P., and S. N. Goodman. 2000. Bayesian communication: a clinically significant paradigm for electronic publication. *Journal of the American Medical Informatics Association* 7:254–266.

Lehmann, H. P., and B. Nguyen. 1997. Bayesian communication of research results over the World Wide Web. *MD Computing* 14:353–359.

Simon, R. M., D. O. Dixon, and B. Freidlin. 1995. A Bayesian model for evaluating specificity of treatment effects in clinical trials. *Cancer Treatment and Research* 75:155–175.

Thall, P. F., and E. H. Estey. 1993. A Bayesian strategy for screening cancer treatments prior to phase II clinical evaluation. *Statistics in Medicine* 12:1197–1211.

Thall, P. F., and R. M. Simon. 1994. Practical Bayesian guidelines for phase II B clinical trials. *Biometrics* 50:337–349.

Thall, P. F., and H. G. Sung. 1998. Some extensions and applications of a Bayesian strategy for monitoring multiple outcomes in clinical trials. *Statistics in Medicine* 17:1563–1580.

Thall, P. F., R. M. Simon, and E. H. Estey. 1995. Bayesian sequential monitoring designs for single-arm clinical trials with multiple outcomes. *Statistics in Medicine* 14:357–379.

Thall, P. F., R. M. Simon, and Y. Shen. 2000. Approximate Bayesian evaluation of multiple treatment effects. *Biometrics* 56:213–219.

Volinsky, C. T., and A. E. Raftery. 2000. Bayesian information criterion for censored survival models. *Biometrics* 56:256–262.

Wakefield, J., and A. Racine-Poon. 1995. An application of Bayesian population pharmacokinetic/pharmacodynamic models to dose determination. *Statistics in Medicine* 14:971–986.

Whitehead, J., and H. Brunier. 1995. Bayesian decision procedures for dose determining experiments. *Statistics in Medicine* 14:885–893.

Whitehead, J., S. Patterson, S. Francis, M. Ireson, and D. Webber. 1999. A novel Bayesian decision procedure for early-phase dose-finding studies. *Journal of Biopharmaceutical Statistics* 9:583–597.

DECISION ANALYSIS

Anis, A. H., P. Tugwell, G. A. Wells, and D. G. Stewart. 1996. A cost-effectiveness analysis of cyclosporine in rheumatoid arthritis. *Journal of Rheumatology* 23:609–616.

Backhouse, M. E. 1998. An investment appraisal approach to clinical trial design. *Health Economics* 7:605–619.

Balas, E. A., R. A. Kretschmer, W. Gnann, D. A. West, S. A. Boren, R. M. Centor, M. Nerlich, M. Gupta, T. D. West, and N. S. Soderstrom. 1998. Interpreting cost analyses of clinical interventions. *Journal of the American Medical Association* 279:54–57.

Berry, D. A., M. C. Wolff, and D. Sack. 1994. Decision making during a phase III randomized controlled trial. *Controlled Clinical Trials* 15:360–378.

Centor, R. M., and J. M. Witherspoon. 1982. Treating sore throats in the emergency room. The importance of follow-up in decision making. *Medical Decision Making* 2:463–469.

Claxton, H. 1999. The irrelevance of inference: a decision-making approach to the stochastic evaluation of health care technologies. *Journal of Health Economics* 18:341–364.

Heitjan, D. F., P. S. Houts, and H. A. Harvey. 1992. A decision-theoretic evaluation of early stopping rules. *Statistics in Medicine* 11:673–683.

Heitjan, D. F., A. J. Moskowitz, and W. Whang. 1999. Bayesian estimation of cost-effectiveness ratios from clinical trials. *Health Economics* 8:191–201.

Heudebert, G. R., R. Marks, C. M. Wilcox, and R. M. Centor. 1997. Choice of long term strategy for the management of patients with severe esophagitis: a cost-utility analysis. *Gastroenterology* 112:1078–1086.

Heudebert, G. R., R. M. Centor, J. C. Klapow, R. Marks, L. Johnson, and C. M. Wilcox. 2000. What is heartburn worth? A cost-utility analysis of management strategies. *Journal of General Internal Medicine* 15:175–182.

Hillner, B. E. and R. M. Centor. 1987. What a difference a day makes: a decision analysis of adult streptococcal pharyngitis. *Journal of General Internal Medicine* 2:244–250.

Huster, W. J., and G. G. Enas. 1998. A framework establishing clear decision criteria for the assessment of drug efficacy. *Statistics in Medicine* 17:1829–1838.

Jonsson, B., and P. E. Bebbington. 1994. What price depression? The cost of depression and the cost-effectiveness of pharmacological treatment. *British Journal of Psychiatry* 164:665–673. (applied decision analysis).

Kattan, M. W., M. E. Cowen, and B. J. Miles. 1997. A decision analysis for treatment of clinically localized prostate cancer. *Journal of General Internal Medicine* 12:299–305.

Mennemeyer, S. T., and L. P. Cyr. 1997. A bootstrap approach to medical decision analysis. *Journal of Health Economics* 16:741–747.

Midgette, A. S., J. B. Wong, J. R. Beshansky, A. Porath, C. Fleming, and S. G. Pauker. 1994. Cost-effectiveness of streptokinase for acute myocardial infarction: a combined meta-analysis and decision analysis of the effects of infarct location and of likelihood of infarction. *Medical Decision Making* 14:108–117.

O'Connor, A. M., P. Tugwell, G. A. Wells, T. Elmslie, E. Jolly, G. Hollingworth, R. McPherson, H. Bunn, I. Graham, and E. Drake. 1998. A decision aid for women considering hormone therapy after menopause: decision support framework and evaluation. *Patient Education Counseling* 33:267–279.

Pliskin, J. S. 1999. Towards better decision making in growth hormone therapy. *Hormone Research* 51(Suppl. 1):30–35.

Samsa, G. P., R. A. Reutter, G. Parmigiani, M. Ancukiewicz, P. Abrahamse, J. Lipscomb, and D. B. Matchar. 1999. Performing cost-effectiveness analysis by integrating randomized trial data with a comprehensive decision model: application to treatment of acute ischemic stroke. *Journal of Clinical Epidemilogy* 52:259–271.

Siegel, J. E., M. C. Weinstein, L. B. Russell, and M. R. Gold. 1996. Recommendations for reporting cost-effectiveness analyses. *Journal of the American Medical Association* 276:1339–1341.

Stallard, N., P. F. Thall, and J. Whitehead. 1999. Decision theoretic designs for phase II clinical trials with multiple outcomes. *Biometrics* 55:971–977.

Stangl, D. K. 1995. Prediction and decision making using Bayesian hierarchical models. *Statistics in Medicine* 14:2173–2190.

Tugwell, P. 1996. Economic evaluation of the management of pain in osteoarthritis. *Drugs* 52(Suppl. 3):48–58.

Tugwell, P., K. J. Bennett, D. L. Sackett, and R. B. Haynes. 1985. The measurement iterative loop: a framework for the critical appraisal of need, benefits and costs of health interventions. *Journal of Chronic Disease* 38:339–351.

Whitehead, J., and H. Brunier. 1995. Bayesian decision procedures for dose determining experiments. *Statistics in Medicine* 14:885-893. (Discussion, 895–899.)

Whitehead, J., and D. Williamson. 1998. Bayesian decision procedures based on logistic regression models for dose-finding studies. *Journal of Biopharmaceutical Statistics* 8: 445–467.

META-ANALYSIS

Aitkin, M. 1999. Meta-analysis by random effect modelling in generalized linear models. *Statistics in Medicine* 18:2343–2351.

Bass, E. B., N. R. Powe, S. N. Goodman, S. L. Graziano, R. I. Griffiths, T. S. Kickler, and J. R. Wingard. 1993. Efficacy of immune globulin in preventing complications of bone marrow transplantation: a meta-analysis. *Bone Marrow Transplant* 12:273–282.

Berkey, C. S., A. Antczak-Bouckoms, D. C. Hoaglin, F. Mosteller, and B. L. Pihlstrom. 1995. Multiple-outcomes meta-analysis of treatments for periodontal disease. *Journal of Dental Research* 74:1030–1039.

Berkey, C. S., D. C. Hoaglin, F. Mosteller, and G. A. Colditz. 1995. A random effects regression model for meta-analysis. *Statistics in Medicine* 14:395–411.

Berkey, C. S., Hoaglin, D. C., A. Antczak-Bouckoms, F. Mosteller, and G. A. Colditz. 1998. Meta-analysis of multiple outcomes by regression with random effects. *Statistics in Medicine* 17:2537–2550.

Boissel, J. P., J. Blanchard, E. Panak, J. C. Peyrieux, and H. Sacks. 1989. Considerations for the meta-analysis of randomized clinical trials. *Controlled Clinical Trials* 10:254–281.

Boutitie, F., F. Gueyffier, S. J. Pocock, and J. P. Boissel.1998. Assessing treatment time interaction in clinical trials with time to event data: a meta-analysis of hypertension trials. *Statistics in Medicine* 17:2883–2903.

Bravata, D. M., I. Olkin, A. E. Barnato, E. B. Keeffe, and D. K. Owens. 1999. Health related quality of life after liver transplantation: a meta-analysis. *Liver Transplant and Surgery* 5:318–331.

Brown, S. A., and L. V. Hedges. 1994. Predicting metabolic control in diabetes: a pilot study using meta-analysis to estimate a linear model. *Nursing Research* 43:362–368.

Brumback, B. A., L. B. Holmes, and L. M. Ryan. 1999. Adverse effects of chorionic villus sampling: a meta-analysis. *Statistics in Medicine* 18:2163–2175.

Bucher, H. C., G. H. Guyatt, L. E. Griffith, and S. D. Walter. 1997. The results of direct and indirect treatment comparisons in meta-analysis of randomized controlled clinical trials. *Journal of Clinical Epidemiology* 50:683–691.

Bucher, H. C., R. J. Cook, G. H. Guyatt, J. D. Lang, D. J. Cook, R. Hatala, and D. L. Hunt. 1996. Effects of dietary calcium supplementation on blood pressure. A meta-analysis of randomized controlled trials. *Journal of the American Medical Association* 275:1016–1022.

Cappelleri, J. C., J. P. Ioannidis, C. H. Schmid, S. D. de Ferranti, M. Aubert, T. C. Chalmers, and J. Lau. 1996. Large trials vs meta-analysis of smaller trials: how do their results compare? *Journal of the American Medical Association* 276:1332–1338.

Christensen, E., and C. Gluud. 1995. Glucocorticoids are ineffective in alcoholic hepatitis: a meta-analysis adjusting for confounding variables. *Gut* 37:113–118.

Cook, R. J., and S. D. Walter 1997. A logistic model for trend in 2 x 2 kappa tables with applications to meta-analysis. *Biometrics* 53:352–357.

Daniels, M. J., and M. D. Hughes. 1997. Meta-analysis for the evaluation of potential surrogate markers. *Statistics in Medicine* 16:1965–1982.

DerSimonian, R. 1996. Meta-analysis in the design and monitoring of clinical trials. *Statistics in Medicine* 15:1237–1248.

Dickersin, K., K. Higgins, and C. L. Meinert. 1990. Identification of meta-analyses. The need for standard terminology. *Controlled Clinical Trials* 11:52–66.

Earle, C. C., B. Pham, and G. A. Wells. 2000. An assessment of methods to combine published survival curves. *Medical Decision Making* 20:104–111.

Egger, M., G. Davey-Smith, C. Stettler, and P. Diem. 1997. Risk of adverse effects of intensified treatment in insulin-dependent diabetes mellitus: a meta-analysis. *Diabetic Medicine* 14:919–928.

Farraz, M. B., P. Tugwell, C. H. Goldsmith, and E. Atra. 1990. Meta-analysis of sulfasalazine in ankolysing spondylitis. *Journal of Rheumatology* 17:1482–1486.

Frost, C., R. Clarke, and H. Beacon. 1999. Use of hierarchical models for meta-analysis: experience in the metabolic ward studies of diet and blood cholesterol. *Statistics in Medicine* 18:1657–1676.

Geller, N. L., and M. Proschan. 1996. Meta-analysis of clinical trials: a consumer's guide. *Journal of Biopharmaceutical Statistics* 6:377–394.

Gloaguen, V., J. Cottraux, M. Cucherat, and I. M. Blackburn. 1998. A meta-analysis of the effects of cognitive therapy in depressed patients. *Journal of Affective Disorder* 49:59–72.

Goodman, S. N. 1989. Meta-analysis and evidence. *Controlled Clinical Trials* 10:188–204.

Goodman, S. N. 1991. Have you ever meta-analysis you didn't like? *Annals of Internal Medicine* 114:244–246.

Hasselblad, V., and D. C. McCrory. 1995. Meta-analytic tools for decision making: a practical guide. *Medical Decision Making* 15:81–96.

Hasselblad, V., and L. V. Hedges. 1995. Meta-analysis of screening and diagnostic tests. *Psychology Bulletin* 117:167–178.

Hauck, W. W., S. Anderson, and S. M. Marcus. 1998. Should we adjust for covariates in nonlinear regression analyses of randomized trials? *Controlled Clinical Trials* 19:249–256.

Hedges, L. V. 1984. Research synthesis: the state of the art. *International Journal of Aging and Human Development* 19:85–93.

Hedges, L. V. 1997. Improving meta-analysis for policy purposes. *NIDA Research Monograph* 170:202–215.

Hendrick, R. E., R. A. Smith, J. H. Rutledge III, and C. R. Smart. 1997. Benefit of screening mammography in women aged 40-49: a new meta-analysis of randomized controlled trials. *Journal of the National Cancer Institute Monograph* 22:87–92.

Higgins, J. P., and A. Whitehead. 1996. Borrowing strength from external trials in a meta-analysis. *Statistics in Medicine* 15:2733–2749.

Homik, J. E., A. Cranney, B. Shea, P. Tugwell, G. Wells, J. D. Adachi, and M. E. Suarez-Almazor. 1999. A meta-analysis on the use of biophosphonates in corticosteroid induced osteoporosis. *Journal of Rheumatology* 26:1148–1157.

Hughes, E. G. 1997. The effectiveness of ovulation induction and intrauterine insemination in the treatment of persistent infertility: a meta-analysis. *Human Reproduction* 12:1865–1872.

Ioannidis, J P., and J. Lau. 1997. The impact of high-risk patients on the results of clinical trials. *Journal of Clinical Epidemiology* 50:1089–1098.

Ioannidis, J. P., and J. Lau. 1998. Heterogeneity of the baseline risk within patient populations of clinical trials: a proposed evaluation algorithm. *American Journal of Epidemiology* 148:1117–1126.

Ioannidis, J. P., J. C. Cappelleri, P. R. Skolnik, J. Lau, and H. S. Sacks. 1996. A meta-analysis of the relative efficacy and toxicity of *Pneumocystis carinii* prophylactic regimens. *Archives of Internal Medicine* 156:177–188.

Jadad, A. R., D. J. Cook, A. Jones, T. P. Klassen, P. Tugwell, M. Moher, and D. Moher. 1998. Methodology and reports of systematic reviews and meta-analyses: a comparison of Cochrane reviews with articles published in paper-based journals. *Journal of the American Medical Association* 280:278–280.

Janicak, P. G., J. M. Davis, R. D. Gibbons, S. Ericksen, S. Chang, and P. Gallagher. 1985. Efficacy of ECT: a meta-analysis. *American Journal of Psychiatry* 142:297–302.

Jones, D. R. 1995. Meta-analysis: weighing the evidence. *Statistics in Medicine* 14:137–149.

Kahn, J. G., B. J. Becker, L. MacIsaa, J. K. Amory, J. Neuhaus, I. Olkin, and M. D. Creinin. 2000. The efficacy of medical abortion: a meta-analysis. *Contraception* 61:29–40.

Karpf, D. B., D. R. Shapiro, E. Seema, K. E. Ensrud, C. C. Jonhston, Jr., S. Adai, S. T. Harris, A. C. Santora II, L. J. Hirsch, L. Oppenheimer, and D. Thompson. 1997. Prevention of nonvertebral fractures by alendronate. A meta-analysis. *Journal of the American Medical Association* 277:1159–1164.

Lau, J., J. P. Ioannidis, and C. H. Schmid.1998. Summing up evidence: one answer is not always enough. *The Lancet* 351:123–127.

Linde, K., N. Clausius, G. Ramirez, D. Melchart, F. Eitel, L. V. Hedges, and W. B. Jonas. 1997. Are the clinical effects of homeopathy placebo effects? A meta-analysis of placebo-controlled trials. *The Lancet* 350:834–843.

Lumley, T., and A. Keech. 1995. Meta-meta-analysis with confidence. *The Lancet* 346:576–577.

Meinert, C. L. 1989. Meta-analysis: science or religion? *Controlled Clinical Trials* 10(4 Suppl.):257S–263S.

Meynaud-Kraemer, L., C. Colin, P. Vergnon, and X. Barth. 1999. Wound infection in open versus laparocopic appendectomy. A meta-analysis. *International Journal of Technology Assessment in Health Care* 15:380–391.

Moher, D., and I. Olkin. 1995. Meta-analysis of randomized controlled trials. A concern for standards. *Journal of the American Medical Association* 274:1962–1964.

Moher, D., B. Pham, A. Jones, D. J. Cook, A. R. Jadad, M. Moher, P. Tugwell, T. P. Klassen. 1998. Does quality of reports of randomised trials affect estimates of intervention efficacy reported in meta-analyses? *The Lancet* 352:609–613.

Moher, D., D. J. Cook, A. R. Jadad, and P. Tugwell, M. Moher, A. Jones, B. Pham, and T. P. Klassen. 1999. Assessing the quality of reports of randomized trials: implications for the conduct of meta-analyses. *Health Technology Assessment* 3:i–iv, 1-98.

Moher, D., D. J. Cook, S. Eastwood, I. Olkin, D. Rennie, and D. F. Stroupe. 1999. Improving the quality of reports of meta-analyses of randomised controlled trials in the QUOROM statement. Quality of reporting of meta-analyses. *The Lancet* 354:1896–1900.

Mushlin, A. I., R. W. Kouides, and D. E. Shapiro. 1998. Estimating the accuracy of screening mammography: a meta-analysis. *American Journal of Preventive Medicine* 14:143–153.

Normand, S. L. 1999. Meta-analysis: formulating, evaluating, combining, and reporting. *Statistics in Medicine* 18:321–359.

Olkin, I. 1994. Re: "A critical look at some popular meta-analytic methods. *American Journal of Epidemiology* 140:297–299. (Discussion, 140:300–301.

Olkin, I. 1995. Meta-analysis: reconciling the results of independent studies. *Statistics in Medicine* 14:457–472.

Olkin, I. 1995. Statistical and theoretical considerations in meta-analysis. *Journal of Clinical Epidemiology* 48:133–146.

Olkin, I. 1996. Meta-analysis: current issues in research synthesis. *Statistics in Medicine* 15:1253–1257.

Olkin, I. 1999. Diagnostic statistical procedures in medical meta-analyses. *Statistics in Medicine* 18:2331–2341.

Olkin, I., and A. Sampson. 1998. Comparison of meta-analysis of variance of individual patient data. *Biometrics* 54:317–322.
Parmar, M. K., L. A. Stewart, and D. G. Altman. 1996. Meta-analyses of randomised trials: when the whole is more than just the sum of the parts. *British Journal of Cancer* 74:496–501.
Parmar, M. K., V. Torri, and L. Stewart. 1998. Extracting summary statistics to perform meta-analyses of the published literature for survival endpoints. *Statistics in Medicine* 17:2815–2834.
Psaty, B. M., N. L. Smith, D. S. Siscovick, T. D. Koepsell, N. S. Weiss, S. R. Heckbert, R. N. Lemaitre, E. H. Wagner, and C. D. Furberg. 1997. Health outcomes associated with anti-hypertensive therapies used as first-line agents. A systematic review and analysis. *Journal of the American Medical Association* 277:739–745.
Rosenthal, R. 1991. *Meta-Analytic Procedures for Social Research. Applied Social Research Methods Series*, Vol. 6. Newbury Park, CA: Sage Publications.
Rothwell, P. M. 1995. Can overall results of clinical trials be applied to all patients? *The Lancet* 345: 1616–1619.
Sankoh, A. J., M. Al-Osh, and M. F. Huque. 1999. On the utility of the Dirichlet distribution for meta-analysis of clinical studies. *Journal of Biopharmaceutical Statistics* 9:289–306.
Schmid, C. H., J. Lau, M. W. McIntosh, and J. C. Cappelleri. 1998. An empirical study of the effect of the control rate as a predictor of treatment efficacy in meta-analysis of clinical trials. *Statistics in Medicine* 17:1923–1942.
Schulz, K. F. 1995. Meta-analyses of interventional trials done in populations with different risks. *The Lancet* 3451304–1305.
Segal, J. B., R. L. McNamara, M. R. Miller, N. Kim, S. N. Goodman, N. R. Powe, K. A. Robinson, and E. B. Bass. 2000. Prevention of thromboembolism in atrial fibrillation. A meta-analysis of trials of anticoagulants and antiplatelet drugs. *Journal of General Internal Medicine* 15:56–67.
Shannon, W. D., and D. Banks. 1999. Combining classification trees using MLE. *Statistics in Medicine* 18:727–740.
Song, F. 1999. Exploring heterogeneity in meta-analysis: is the L'Abbe plot useful? *Journal of Clinical Epidemiology* 52:725–730.
Steinberg, K. K., S. B. Thacker, S. J. Smith, D. F. Stroup, M. M. Zack, W. D. Flanders, and R. L. Berkelman. 1991. A meta-analysis of the effect of estrogen replacement therapy on the risk of breast cancer. *Journal of the American Medical Association* 265:1985–1990.
Steinberg, K. K., S. J. Smith, D. F. Stroup, I. Olkin, N. C. Lee, G. D. Williamson, and S. B. Thacker. 1997. Comparison of effect estimates from a meta-analysis of summary data from published studies and from a meta-analysis using individual patient data for ovarian cancer studies. *American Journal of Epidemiology* 145:917–925.
Stijnen, T. 2000. Tutorial in biostatistics. Meta-analysis: formulating, evaluating, combining, and reporting by S. L. Normand (letter). *Statistics in Medicine* 19:759–761.
Stram, D. O. 1996. Meta-analysis of published data using a linear mixed-effects model. *Biometrics* 52:536–544.
Stroup, D. F., J. A. Berlin, S. C. Morton, I. Olkin, G. D. Williamson, D. Rennie, D. Moher, B. J. Becker, T. A. Sipe, and S. B. Thacker. 2000. Meta-analysis of

observational studies in epidemiology: a proposal for reporting. Meta-analysis of Observational Studies in Epidemiology (MOOSE) Group. *Journal of the American Medical Association* 283:2008–2012.

Szczech, L. A., J. A. Berlin, S. Aradhye, R. A. Grosman, and H. I. Feldman. 1997. Effect of anti-lymphocyte induction therapy on renal allograft survival: a meta-analysis. *Journal of the American Society of Nephrology* 8:1771–1777.

Thacker, S. B., D. F. Stroup, and H. B. Peterson. 1998. Meta-analysis for the practicing obstetrician-gynecologist. *Clinical Obstetrics and Gynecology* 41:275–281.

Thompson, S. G., and S. J. Sharp. 1999. Explaining heterogeneity in meta-analysis: a comparison of methods. *Statistics in Medicine* 18:2693–2708.

Thompson, S. G., T. C. Smith, and S. J. Sharp. 1997. Investigating underlying risk as a source of heterogeneity in meta-analysis. *Statistics in Medicine* 16:2741–2758.

Tugwell, P. 1996. Combination therapy in rheumatoid arthritis: meta-analysis. *Journal of Rheumatology* 44(Suppl.):43-46.

Whitehead, A. 1997. A prospectively planned cumulative meta-analysis applied to a series of concurrent clinical trials. *Statistics in Medicine* 16:2901–2913.

Whitehead, A., A. J. Bailey, and D. Elbourne. 1999. Combining summaries of binary outcomes with those of continuous outcomes in a meta-analysis. *Journal of Biopharmaceutical Statistics* 9:1–16.

Whitehead, J., and A. Whitehead. 1991. A general parametric approach to the meta-analysis of randomized clinical trials. *Statistics in Medicine* 10:1665–1677.

META-ANALYSIS, CONFIDENCE PROFILE METHOD

Ananth, C. V., and J. S. Preisser. 1999. Bivariate logistic regression: modelling the association of small for gestational age births in twin gestations. *Statistics in Medicine* 18: 2011–2023.

Eddy, D. M., V. Hasselblad, and R. Schacter. 1990. An introduction to a Bayesian method for meta-analysis: the confidence profile method. *Medical Decision Making* 10:15–23.

Eddy, D. M., V. Hasselblad, and R. Shachter. 1992. *Meta-Analysis by the Confidence Profile Method. The Statistical Synthesis of Evidence.* Boston: Academic Press, Inc./ Harcourt Brace Jovanovich, Publishers.

Hardy, R. J., and S. G. Thompson. 1996. A likelihood approach to meta-analysis with random effects. *Statistics in Medicine* 15:619–629.

Hardy, R. J., and S. G. Thompson. 1998. Detecting and describing heterogeneity in meta-analysis. *Statistics in Medicine* 17:841–856.

N-OF-1 CLINICAL TRIALS

Cook, D. J. 1996. Randomized trials in single subjects: the *n*-of-1 study. *Psychopharmacology Bulletin* 32:363–367.

Edgington, E. S. 1996. Randomized single-subject experimental designs. *Behaviour Research and Therapy* 34:567–574.

Fleming, T. R. 1982. One-sample multiple testing procedure for phase II clinical trials. *Biometrics* 38:143–151.

Frasca, M. A., and J. C. Aldag. 1988. The single-patient clinical trial. *American Family Physician* 37:195–199.

Guyatt, G. H., D. Sackett, J. Adachi, R. Roberts, J. Chong, D. Rosenbloom, and J. Keller. 1988. A clinician's guide for conducting randomized trials in individual patients. *Canadian Medical Association Journal* 139:497–503.

Hodgson, M. 1993. *n*-of-1 clinical trials. The practice of environmental and occupational medicine. *Journal of Occupational Medicine* 35:375–380.

Johannessen, T. 1991. Controlled trials in single subjects. 1. Value in clinical medicine. *British Medical Journal* 303:173–174.

Johannessen, T., D. Fosstvedt, and H. Petersen. 1988. Experience with multi-crossover model in dyspepsia. *Scandinavian Journal of Gastroenterology Supplement* 147:33–37.

Johannessen, T., D. Fosstvedt, and H. Petersen. 1990. Statistical aspects of controlled single subject trials. *Family Practice* 7:325–328.

Johannessen, T., D. Fosstvedt, and H. Petersen. 1991. Combined single subject trials. *Scandinavian Journal of Primary Health Care* 9:23–27.

Johannessen, T., H. Petersen, P. Kristensen, and D. Fosstvedt. 1991. The controlled single subject trial. *Scandinavian Journal of Primary Health Care* 9:17–21.

Johannessen, T., P. Kirsten, H. Petersen, D. Fosstvedt, I. Loge, P. M. Kleveland, and J. Dybdahl. 1991. The symptomatic effect of 1-day treatment periods with cimetidine in dyspepsia. Combined results from randomized, controlled, single-subject trials. *Scandinavian Journal of Gastroenterology* 26:974–980.

Keller, J. L., G. H. Guyatt, R. S. Robarts, J. D. Adachi, and D. Rosenbloom. 1988. An *n*-of-1 service: applying the scientific method in clinical practice. *Scandinavian Journal of Gastroenterology Supplement* 147:22–29.

Lewis, J. A. 1991. Controlled trials in single subjects. 2. Limitations of use. *British Medical Journal* 303:175–176.

Lindberg, G. 1988. Single case studies in clinical trials. *Scandinavian Journal of Gastroenterology Supplement* 147:30–32.

Lukoff, D., D. Edwards, and M. Miller. 1998. The case study as a scientific method for researching alternative therapies. *Alternative Therapies in Health Medicine* 4:44–52.

Menard, J., M. Bellet, and D. Serrurier. 1990. From the parallel group design to the crossover design, and from the group approach to the individual approach. *American Journal of Hypertension* 3:815–819.

Morley, S., and M. Adams. 1989. Some simple statistical tests for exploring single-case time-series data. *British Journal of Clinical Psychology* 28 (Pt 1):1–18.

O'Brien, P. C. 1997. The use and misuse of *n*-of-1 studies (editorial). *International Journal of Oral and Maxillofacial Implants* 12:293.

Sandvik, L. 1988. Single case studies from a statistician's point of view. *Scandinavian Journal of Gastroenterology Supplement* 147:38–39.

Sjoden, P. O. 1988. Single case studies in psychology and psychiatry. *Scandinavian Journal of Gastroenterology Supplement* 147:11–21.

Spiegelhalter, D. J. 1988. Statistical issues in studies of individual response. *Scandinavian Journal of Gastroenterology Supplement* 147:40–45.

Treasure, W. 1996. N-of-1 trials. Placebos should be abandoned. *British Medical Journal* 313: 427–428.

Whitehead, J., W. M. Gregory, K. Bolland, and R. L. Souhami. 1997. Cautionary tales of survival analysis: conflicting analyses from a clinical trial in breast cancer. *British Journal of Cancer* 76:551–558.

Wulff, H. R. 1988. Single case studies: an introduction. *Scandinavian Journal of Gastroenterology Supplement* 147:7–10.

Zucker, D. R., C. H. Schmid, M. W. McIntosh, R. B. D'Agostino, H. P. Selker, and J. Lau. 1997. Combining single patient trials to estimate population treatment effects and to evaluate individual patient responses to treatment. *Journal of Clinical Epidemiology* 50:401–410.

SEQUENTIAL ANALYSIS

Armitage, P. 1975. *Sequential Medical Trials.* New York: Wiley.

Atkinson, A. C. 1999. Optimum biased-coin designs for sequential treatment allocation with covariate information. *Statistics in Medicine* 18:1741–1752. (Discussion, 18:1753–1755.)

Bellissant, E., J. Benichou, and C. Chastang. 1996. The group sequential triangular test for phase II cancer clinical trials. *American Journal of Clinical Oncology* 19:422–430.

Betensky, R. A. 1997. Conditional power calculations for early acceptance of H_o embedded in sequential tests. *Statistics in Medicine* 16:465–477.

Brooks, M. M., A. Hallstrom, and M. Peckova. 1995. A simulation study used to design the sequential monitoring plan for a clinical trial. *Statistics in Medicine* 14:2227–2237.

Carlin, B. P., J. B. Kadane, and A. E. Gelfand. 1998. Approaches for optimal sequential decision analysis in clinical trials. *Biometrics* 54:964–975.

Conoway, M. R. and G. R. Petroni. 1996. Designs for phase II trials allowing for a trade-off between response and toxicity. *Biometrics* 52:1375–1386. (applied sequential methods)

DeMets, D. L. 1989. Group sequential procedures: calendar versus information time. *Statistics in Medicine* 8:1191–1198.

DeMets, D. L. and G. Lan. 1995. The alpha spending function approach to interim data analyses. *Cancer Treatment and Research* 75:1–27.

DeMets, D. L., D. Y. Lin, and L. J. Wei. 1991. Exact statistical inference for group sequential trials. *Biometrics* 47:1399–1408.

Emerson, S. S. 1995. Stopping a clinical trial very early based on unplanned interim analyses: a group sequential approach. *Biometrics* 51:1152–1162.

Emerson, S. S., and T. R. Fleming. 1989. Symmetric group sequential test designs. *Biometrics* 45:905–923.

Emerson, S. S., and T. R. Fleming. 1990. Interim analyses in clinical trials. *Oncology* 4:126–133. (Discussion, 4:134, 136.)

Fleming, T. R., D. P. Harrington, and P. C. O'Brien. 1984. Designs for group sequential tests. *Controlled Clinical Trials* 5:348–361.

Geller, N. L., and Z. H. Li. 1991. On the choice of times for data analysis in group sequential clinical trials. *Biometrics* 47:745–750.

Hallstrom, A., R. McBride, and R. Moore. 1995. Toward vital status sweeps: a case history in sequential monitoring. *Statistics in Medicine* 14:1927–1931.

Heitjan, D. F. 1997. Bayesian interim analysis of phase II cancer clinical trials. *Statistics in Medicine* 16:1791–1802.

Jiang, W. 1999. Group sequential procedures for repeated events data with frailty. *Journal of Biopharmaceutical Statistics* 9:379–399.

Kim, K., and D. L. DeMets.1987. Confidence intervals following group sequential tests in clinical trials. *Biometrics* 43:857–864.

Lai, T. L., B. Levin, H. Robbins, and D. Siegmund. 1980. Sequential medical trials. *Proceedings of the National Academy of Sciences USA* 77:3135–3138.

Lan, K. K., and D. L. DeMets. 1989. Changing frequency of interim analysis in sequential monitoring. *Biometrics* 45:1017–1020.

Lan, K. K., W. F. Rosenberger, and J. M. Lachin. 1995. Sequential monitoring of survival data with the Wilcoxon statistic. *Biometrics* 51:1175–1183.

Lee, J. W., and D. L. DeMets. 1995. Group sequential comparison of changes: ad-hoc versus more exact method. *Biometrics* 51:21–30.

Lee, J. W., and H. N. Sather. 1995. Group sequential methods for comparison of cure rates in clinical trials. *Biometrics* 51:756–763.

Liu, W. 1995. A group sequential procedure for all pairwise comparisons of k treatments based on the range statistic. *Biometrics* 51:946–955.

O'Fallon, J. R. 1985. Policies for interim analysis and interim reporting of results. *Cancer Treatment Reports* 69:1101–1116.

O'Quigley, J., and L. Z. Shen. 1996. Continual reassessment method: a likelihood approach. *Biometrics* 52:673–684.

Pocock, S. J., and M. D. Hughes. 1989. Practical problems in interim analyses, with particular regard to estimation. *Controlled Clinical Trials* 10(Suppl.):209S–221S.

Reboussin D. M., D. L. DeMets, K. Kim, and K. K. Lan. 2000. Computations for group sequential boundaries using the Lan-DeMets spending function method. *Controlled Clinical Trials* 21:190–207.

Tan, M., and X. Xiong. 1996. Continuous and group sequential conditional probability ratio tests for phase II clinical trials. *Statistics in Medicine* 15:2037–2051.

Tan, M., X. Xiong, and M. H. Kutner. 1998. Clinical trial designs based on sequential conditional probability ratio tests and reverse stochastic curtailing. *Biometrics* 54(2):682-695.

Whitehead, J. 1986. Supplementary analysis at the conclusion of a sequential clinical trial. *Biometrics* 42:461–471.

Whitehead, J. 1991. Four problems with group sequential methods. *Controlled Clinical Trials* 12:340–344.

Whitehead, J. 1992. Overrunning and underrunning in sequential clinical trials. *Controlled Clinical Trials* 13:106–121.

Whitehead, J. 1993. Interim analyses and stopping rules in cancer clinical trials. *British Journal of Cancer* 68:1179–1185.

Whitehead, J. 1994. Sequential methods based on the boundaries approach for the clinical comparison of survival times. *Statistics in Medicine* 13:1357–1368. (Discussion 1369–1370.)

Whitehead, J. 1997. *The Design and Analysis of Sequential Clinical Trials.* New York: Ellis Horwood.

Whitehead, J. 1998. Sequential designs for equivalence studies. *Statistics in Medicine* 15:2703–2715.

Whitehead, J. 1999. A unified theory for sequential clinical trials. *Statistics in Medicine* 18: 2271–2286.

Whitehead, J., and K. M. Facey. 1990. An improved approximation for calculation of confidence intervals after a sequential clinical trial. *Statistics in Medicine* 9:1277–1285.

Whitehead, J., and K. M. Facey. 1990. The impact that group sequential tests would have made on ECOG clinical trials. *Statistics in Medicine* 9:853–854.

Whitehead, J., and D. R. Jones. 1979. Group sequential methods. *British Journal of Cancer* 40:171–172.

Whitehead, J., and P. Marek. 1985. A Fortran program for the design and analysis of sequential clinical trials. *Computers and Biomedical Research* 18:176–183.

Whitehead, J., and M. R. Sooriyarachchi. 1998. A method for sequential analysis of survival data with non-proportional hazards. *Biometrics* 54:1072–1084.

Whitehead, J., and I. Stratton. 1983. Group sequential clinical trials with triangular continuation regions. *Biometrics* 39:227–236.

Whitehead, J., and P. Thomas. 1997. A sequential trial of painkillers in arthritis: issues of multiple comparisons with control and of interval-censored survival data. *Journal of Biopharmaceutical Statistics* 7:333–353.

Whitehead, J., D. R. Jones, and C. E. Newman. 1982. The design of a sequential clinical trial for the comparison of two lung cancer treatments. *Statistics in Medicine* 1:73–82.

Whitehead, J., D. R. Jones, and S. H. Ellis. 1983. The analysis of a sequential clinical trial for the comparison of two lung cancer treatments. *Statistics in Medicine* 2:183–190.

Whitehead, J., A. N. Donaldson, R. Stephens, and D. Machin. 1993. A simulated sequential analysis based on data from two MRC trials. *British Journal of Cancer* 68:1171–1178.

Williams, P. L. 1996. Sequential monitoring of clinical trials with multiple survival endpoints. *Statistics in Medicine* 15:2341–2357.

Appendix D
Committee and Staff Biographies

COMMITTEE BIOGRAPHIES

Robert M. Centor, M.D., is professor of medicine, director of the Division of General Internal Medicine, and associate dean for Primary Care and Continuing Medical Education at the University of Alabama School of Medicine. Dr. Centor maintains an active interest in medical decision making, cost-effectiveness analysis, and outcomes research.

Ed Davis, Ph.D., is the chairman of the Department of Biostatistics in the School of Public Health at the University of North Carolina Chapel Hill. He received a Ph.D. in experimental statistics from North Carolina State University. He is an applied statistician with research interests in the design, conduct, and analysis of data from clinical trials and prospective epidemiological studies. His statistical research is in nonparametric methods.

Suzanne T. Ildstad, M.D., is a specialist in small-number-participant clinical trials, director of the Institute for Cellular Therapeutics, and The Jewish Hospital Distinguished Professor of Transplantation and Surgery at the University of Louisville. Dr. Ildstad received a medical degree from the Mayo Medical School in Rochester, Minnesota, followed by a residency in general surgery at the Massachusetts General Hospital, an immunology fellowship at the National Institutes of Health, and a pediatric surgery-transplant surgery fellowship in Cincinnati. Her research in mixed chimerism to induce tolerance to organ allografts and treat nonmalignant diseases such as sickle cell anemia and autoimmune disorders is being applied clinically in six Food and Drug Administration-approved phase I trials. Dr. Ildstad holds several patents related to her research in expanding bone marrow transplantation to treat nonmalignant disease by optimizing the risk-benefit ratio through graft engineering and partial conditioning. She is the founding scientist of Chimeric Therapies, Inc., a biotechnology company focused on bone marrow graft engineering, and she serves on the board of directors of the company. Dr. Ildstad is a member of the Institute of Medicine, is serving as correspondent for the Committee on Human Rights, and is a member of the Institute of Medicine Committees on Organ Procurement and Transplantation and Multiple Sclerosis: Current Status and Strategies for the Future.

Bruce Levin, Ph.D., is professor and head of the Division of Biostatistics at the Columbia School of Public Health. He received a Ph.D. from Harvard University and has been on the faculty at Columbia University since 1974. His research interests are in biostatistics, data analysis, logistic regression, and sequential analysis. He is principal investigator of the Statistics, Epidemiology, and Data Management Core of the HIV Center for Clinical and Behavioral Studies. He is the senior statistical consultant on several multicenter randomized clinical trials in the field of stroke neurology and cardiology, including the Warfarin and Aspirin Recurrent Stroke Study and its collaborative trials. Dr. Levin has also served for the past 8 years as a consulting statistical editor for the *American Journal of Public Health*. He has a long-standing interest in the intersection of statistical inference for categorical data and computational methods in statistics. This interest has resulted in the development of analytical methods for a variety of problems from a unified viewpoint (that of finite and infinite dimensional linear exponential families). A product of this work is the unique computing program MCLA for maximum conditional likelihood analysis of polytomous outcome data in large-scale epidemiological data sets with arbitrary levels of stratification. Dr. Levin also studies general empirical Bayes methods (e.g., to test homogeneity hypotheses in large sparse data sets). Using these methods, Dr. Levin explores alternative designs for clinical trials, including nonrandomized designs that ensure allocation of new treatment to those subjects in most dire need of therapy. A related area of interest is sequential trial design, both classical and innovative (e.g., designs that minimize ethical costs).

Edward D. Miller, M.D., was named chief executive officer of Johns Hopkins Medicine, the 13th dean of The Johns Hopkins University School of Medicine, and vice president for medicine of The Johns Hopkins University in January 1997. He received an A.B. from Ohio Wesleyan University and an M.D. from the University of Rochester School of Medicine and Dentistry. He was a surgical intern at University Hospital in Boston, chief resident in anesthesiology at Peter Bent Brigham Hospital in Boston, and a research fellow in physiology at the Harvard Medical School. In 1981–1982, he spent a sabbatical year as senior scientist at Hôpital Necker in Paris. He joined Hopkins in 1994 as professor and chairman of the Department of Anesthesiology and Critical Care Medicine, a post he held until May 1999. He was named interim dean of the School of Medicine in 1996. He came to Hopkins after 8 years at Columbia University in New York, where he served as professor and chairman of the Department of Anesthesiology in the College of Physicians and Surgeons. Before that he spent 11 years at the University of Virginia in Charlottesville, where he rose from assistant professor to professor of anesthesiology and surgery and medical director of the Surgical Intensive Care Unit. Dr. Miller's research has focused on the cardiovascular effects of anesthetic drugs and vascular smooth muscle relaxation. He has served as president of the Association of University Anesthesiologists and editor of *Anesthesia and Analgesia* and of *Critical Care Medicine*. Elected to the Royal College of Anaesthetists in London in 1993, he has served on the board of the International Anesthesia Research Society and from 1991 to 1994 was chair of the Food and Drug Administration's Advisory Committee on Anesthesia and Life Support Drugs. A member of the Institute of Medicine of the National Academy of Sciences, Dr. Miller has authored or co authored more than 150 scientific papers, abstracts, and book chapters.

Ingram Olkin, Ph.D., is professor of statistics and education at Stanford University. He received a doctorate in mathematical statistics from the University of North Carolina and before moving to Stanford was on the faculties of Michigan State University and the University of Minnesota, where he served as chair of the Department of Statistics. He has co written a number of books, including *Inequalities: Theory of Majorization and its Applications* (1979), *Selecting and Ordering Populations* (1980), *Probability Models and Applications* (1980), and most recently, *Statistical Methods in Meta-Analysis* (1985). Dr. Olkin has been an editor of the *Annals of Statistics* and an associate editor of *Psychometrika*, the *Journal of Educational Statistics*, and the *Journal of the American Statistical Association*. He has also served as chair of the Committee of Applied and Theoretical Statistics, National Research Council, National Academy of Sciences, and president of the Institute of Mathematical Statistics. He has been an Overseas Fellow, Churchill College, Cambridge University; a Lady Davis Fellow, Hebrew University; an Alexander von Humboldt Fellow, University of Augsburg; and a Guggenheim Fellow. He received an honorary D.Sci from DeMontfort University; a Lifetime Contribution Award from the American Psychological Association, Division 5; and a Wilks Medal from the American Statistical Association. His recent interest has been methodology for research synthesis, and he has published both theoretical and applied papers in medicine. He is currently a fellow in the Primary Care Outcomes Research program. His work in meta-analysis was the subject of his R.A. Fisher Lecture at the Joint Statistical Meeting 2000.

David J. Tollerud, M.D., M.P.H., is professor of public health at the MCP Hahnemann University School of Public Health. He received an M.D. from Mayo Medical School and an M.P.H. from the Harvard School of Public Health. He served as a medical staff fellow in the Environmental Epidemiology Branch, National Cancer Institute; pulmonary fellow at Brigham and Women's and Beth Israel Hospitals in Boston; assistant professor of medicine at the University of Cincinnati; and associate professor of environmental and occupational health at the University of Pittsburgh Graduate School of Public Health. He is a fellow of the American College of Occupational and Environmental Medicine and the American College of Chest Physicians; a member of numerous professional societies, including the American Thoracic Society, the American Association of Immunologists, the Clinical Immunology Society, the American Public Health Association, and the American Association for the Advancement of Science; and a member of the editorial review board of the *American Industrial Hygiene Association Journal.*

Peter Tugwell, M.D., M.Sc., is professor and chair of the Department of Medicine at the University of Ottawa. He received an M.D. from the University of London. From 1979 to 1991 he was chair of the Department of Epidemiology and Biostatistics at McMaster University, and from 1987 to 1991 he was director of the McMaster Rheumatology Program/The Centre for Arthritic Diseases. He joined the University of Ottawa as chair of the Department of Medicine and as physician-in-chief at the Ottawa General Hospital in July 1991. Since coming to Ottawa he has been an investigator in the Loeb/University of Ottawa Clinical Epidemiology Unit. Dr. Tugwell was awarded the 1997 Researcher of the Year Award from the Ottawa General Hospital. He has been actively involved in several international organizations. He was the founding director of the McMaster Training Centre for the International Clinical Epidemiology Network (INCLEN) from 1980 to 1991 and recently has served as Chair of the INCLEN Research Subcommittee. He was president of the Canadian Society for International Health from 1989 to 1991. Dr. Tugwell is currently director of the World Health Organization Collaborating Centre for Health Technology Assessment based in Ottawa. He is the author or coauthor of more than 260 published articles. His research interests are in rheumatology, cytokines, and health technology assessment.

HEALTH SCIENCES POLICY BOARD LIAISON

Robert Gibbons, Ph.D., is professor of biostatistics and director of the Center for Health Statistics at the University of Illinois at Chicago. He received his doctorate in statistics and psychometrics from the University of Chicago in 1981. In 1985 he received a young scientist award from the Office of Naval Research, which funded his statistical research in the areas of the analysis of multivariate binary data and the analysis of longitudinal data. Dr. Gibbons has also received additional grant support from the National Institutes of Health and the John D. and Catherine T. MacArthur Foundation. He currently has a research scientist award from the National Institutes of Health that provides full-time support for statistical research. Applications of Dr. Gibbons' work are widespread in the general areas of mental health and environmental sciences. Dr. Gibbons has authored more than 100 peer-reviewed scientific papers and two books. He is currently working on a book entitled *Statistical Methods for Detection and Quantification of Environmental Contamination*, which will be published by John Wiley & Sons. He served on the Institute of Medicine's Committee on Halcion: An Assessment of Data Adequacy and Confidence as well as the Institute of Medicine's Committee on Organ Procurement and Transplantation Policy. Dr. Gibbons also is a member of the Health Sciences Policy Board of the Institute of Medicine.

IOM STUDY STAFF BIOGRAPHIES

Charles H. Evans, Jr., M.D., Ph.D., is Senior Adviser for Biomedical and Clinical Research at the Institute of Medicine of the National Academies. A pediatrician and immunologist, he graduated with a B.S. in biology from

Union College and an M.D. and a Ph.D. from the University of Virginia and trained in pediatrics at the University of Virginia Medical Center. From 1975 to 1998 he served as chief of the Tumor Biology Section at the National Cancer Institute and holds the rank of Captain (Ret.) in the U.S. Public Health Service with 27 years of service as a medical scientist at the National Institutes of Health in Bethesda, Maryland. Dr. Evans' research interests include carcinogenesis (the etiology of cancer), the normal immune system defenses to the development of cancer, and aerospace medicine. He discovered the ability of cytokines to directly prevent carcinogenesis and was the first to isolate a direct-acting anticarcinogenic cytokine for which he was awarded four U.S. patents. Dr. Evans is the author of more than 125 scientific articles and is the recipient of numerous scientific awards including the Outstanding Service Medal from the U.S. Public Health Service and the Wellcome Medal and Prize. He is a fellow of the American Association for the Advancement of Science, a fellow of the American Institute of Chemists, and a credentialed Fellow in Health Systems Administration of the American Academy of Medical Administrators. An active adviser to community medicine and higher education, he has served on the Board of Trustees of Suburban Hospital Health System and on the College of Arts & Sciences Board of Trustees at the University of Virginia. Dr. Evans is the study director for the Committee on Strategies for Small-Number-Participant Clinical Research Trials.

Veronica A. Schreiber, M.A., M.P.H., received an M.P.H. with concentration in epidemiology from the George Washington University in 1999. For her master's research project, she designed and conducted research on patient referral and consultation practices by physicians of the Ambulatory Care Department of the George Washington University Medical Center. Before her health research work, she held teaching positions in political science and international relations for 11 years at the University of the Philippines (1974 to 1980), University of Pittsburgh (1980 to 1983), Frostburg State University (1983 to 1984), and the University of Maryland European Division (1988 to 1989). She was a Ph.D. candidate at the University of Pittsburgh when she accepted a teaching position at Frostburg State University in 1983. She was a research consultant at the Bonn office of the European Institute for Environmental Policy (1987 to 1988) and a training specialist at the German Foundation for International Development (1988 to 1991). She is a member of the Pi Sigma Alpha (political science) National Honor Society and the Phi Theta Kappa International Honor Society. After several years of community volunteer work and as a full-time mother, Ms.

Schreiber joined the Institute of Medicine as the research assistant for the Committee on Strategies for Small-Number-Participant Clinical Research Trials and the Committee on Creating a Vision for Space Medicine Beyond Earth Orbit.

Kathi E. Hanna, Ph.D., is a science and health policy consultant specializing in biomedical research policy, specifically, genetics, cancer, and reproductive technologies. Most recently, Dr. Hanna served as senior adviser to the National Bioethics Advisory Commission in its response to the president's request for recommendations regarding human cloning. Before that she was senior adviser to the President's Advisory Committee on Gulf War Veterans Illnesses, in which she assessed the effects of military service on the reproductive health of veterans. Dr. Hanna was a senior analyst at the congressional Office of Technology Assessment for 7 years and contributed to numerous science policy studies requested by committees of the U.S. Congress on biotechnology, human genetics, women's health, reproductive technologies, and bioethics. In 1989, Dr. Hanna spent a year at the Institute of Medicine, where she edited a book about the interface between biomedical research and politics. In the past decade, Dr. Hanna has also served as a consultant to the Howard Hughes Medical Institute, the National Institutes of Health, the Institute of Medicine, the Federation of American Societies of Experimental Biology, and several academic health centers. Before her work in Washington, D.C., Dr. Hanna was the genetics coordinator at Children's Memorial Hospital in Chicago. Dr. Hanna received an A.B. in biology from Lafayette College, an M.S. in human genetics from Sarah Lawrence College, and a doctorate from the School of Business and Public Management, George Washington University.

Tanya Lee is project assistant for the Small Clinical Trials Study and the Space Medicine Study in the Board of Health Science Policy of the Institute of Medicine. She has been with the National Academies since April 2000. Ms. Lee attended the University of Maryland Eastern Shore and Prince Georges Community College, pursuing a degree in the field of sociology.